THE TWO MARTINI DIET

Also by Jerry Sorlucco

A Good Stick
An Airline Captain Lives the History of 20th Century Commercial Aviation

Facing Fascism
The Threat to American Democracy in the 21st Century

The Two Martini Diet

How I Lost 100+lbs While Eating Well and Having a Drink

by

Jerry Sorlucco

authorHOUSE®

AuthorHouse™
1663 Liberty Drive, Suite 200
Bloomington, IN 47403
www.authorhouse.com
Phone: 1-800-839-8640

First published by AuthorHouse 11/12/2008

ISBN: 978-1-4389-2084-9 (e)
ISBN: 978-1-4389-2083-2 (sc)

Library of Congress Control Number: 2008910346

Printed in the United States of America
Bloomington, Indiana

This book is printed on acid-free paper.

To
My wife Sue,
Whose support made it all a piece of cake

TABLE OF CONTENTS

INTRODUCTION

Jerry Sorlucco, author of *The Two Martini Diet*, has broken new ground in the war against obesity and the serious, chronic health problems that being overweight can bring. He is not a dietitian, food guru, chef or any other type of food expert who just gives advice. He practices what he preaches. He's lost over 100 pounds in about 2 years and I have seen the before and after in person. *The Two Martini Diet* is not really like the typical diet book – 50 or fewer pages of information and 200 pages of recipes. There are no recipes in his book, that is, aside from a few of his favorite meals and how to make a really good martini. What there is in place of recipes is a very thorough and thoughtful investigation of food and its manufacture.

Yes, as Jerry points out, it's the manufactured foods with high fructose corn syrup and CAFOs (Consolidated Animal Feeding Operations) that are killing us. More veggies and fiber promote good health and good body function. But you have to know that a diet consisting largely of veggies and fiber leads to more hunger if you are burning (fat) calories. You will have to eat more frequently because veggies and fiber contain few calories. Once you have burned all your fat, you will have to eat some carbohydrate for energy and to maintain the weight that makes you feel good. You also have to eat protein, preferably from grass-fed beef, poultry and pork and dairy products such as eggs.

If you have ever been very overweight and lost that weight through improved eating habits (notice I did not say 'diet') and exercise, you can easily recall how poorly you felt when overweight and how wonderful you felt without the excess.

The *Two Martini Diet* also tells us that all fat is not bad for you and all fat is not just fat. Fish, in particular, is loaded with fat, but fat that is really good for you. Cardiologists now prescribe fish oil capsules that contain good fats for people who have had heart attacks. The good fats in fish and fish oil promote blood thinning and healthy blood vessels that do not clog up (atherosclerosis) and cause blood to clot (thrombosis) which can lead to a heart attack, stroke or other catastrophe.

I am a physician with over 35 years of experience counseling patients to eat less and exercise more. But I also fell victim to the first U.S. Department of Agriculture Food Pyramid. Despite jogging 6 to 12 miles a week to stay fit and keep my weight down and eating more pasta, bread, rice and less meat and fat as the pyramid dictated, I ballooned from 190 to 225 pounds. As a physician I am supposed to know about nutrition. Obviously I didn't know enough to help myself, let alone any patients.

Thanks to *The Two Martini Diet*, which brings together important information from many sources into one delightful, and easy to read book, I, too, am winning my own personal war with weight, energy level and sense of well-being? And I am recommending Jerry's book to anyone who laments their inability to take off pounds.

The *Two Martini Diet* emphasizes repeatedly that more calories (more food) eaten than burned causes weight gain. And more calories burned than eaten (less food) causes weight loss. This is an indisputable fact, a law of nature if you will. Using prescription and non-prescription drugs or believing media hype that lets you lose weight while you sleep or eat anything and/or as much of anything you want and still lose weight is just, well, plain crap.

There is one important benefit of eating less food. Your stomach shrinks (yes, it really does!). Then you know if you eat too much, because it hurts when stretched. This is called positive feedback. The pain reminds you not to eat so much.

Another useful tip to win the weight war: eat only when you are hungry, not when the TV ads or the McDonald's, Burger King, Pizza

Hut, Quizzno's sign tells you that you are hungry and invites you to eat. There is no rule that says you have to eat three or more meals daily.

Finishing the *Two Martini Diet* should not be the goal or end of the reason you bought this book, but the beginning of your own personal and successful journey to eat well, enjoy a good martini (or a diet soda with a splash of maraschino cherry juice), feel better, live healthier and longer in good health.

Robert A. Peraino, M.D.

PREFACE

In 2006, at the age of sixty-nine, following arthroscopic surgery to clean out a bum knee, I faced a choice. Lose weight or plan on knee replacements. My weight had drifted north since retiring as an airline captain nine years before, and at five-foot nine I grossed two-hundred seventy-pounds, my highest weight ever. And it wasn't only my knee that was bothering me: I suffered frequent sciatica (sharp pain through the lower back and buttocks), foot arch pain, high blood pressure, sleep-apnea (the sleep clinic found I was waking up once a minute for lack of air), a herniated belly button (caused by the stress of a fifty-four inch belly), erectile dysfunction (for the first time in my life), and was diagnosed with low testosterone (a male hormone deficiency). Clearly, if I wanted to continue doing the things I enjoy and live into a healthy old age, I had to lose weight.

I did, and I now weigh 168 pounds, down from 270—over one hundred pounds in twenty-four months, an average of a pound a week. And I feel and look great! I went from a size fifty-four waist and jacket size—a square sort of shape—to a size forty-two jacket and a thirty-seven waist. Yes, once again I have a waist, and my pants stay up. Nothing hurts, I don't get winded going up stairs (or enjoying sex), my sleep apnea is gone, along with the controlled positive air pressure (CPAP) mask I'd been forced to sleep with for years, and my blood pressure and cholesterol levels are well within the normal to excellent range.

When I run into people I haven't seen for some time, the response is funny. First the concerned look and then the question, "Are you feeling all right?" Basically they are asking what dread disease I'm dying of. When told the story, their next question is how in the world did you do it? Not surprising, two-thirds of the adults in America are either overweight or obese, and like as not they're fighting to lose weight themselves. This book is an effort to answer that question. "How did I do it?" The answer is both amazingly simple and extremely complex.

Simply, one gets overweight by eating more food calories (energy) than the body can use, which is then stored as fat. If energy in is equal to energy out, you maintain weight. Eat more than you burn and you gain weight. Reverse the process and you lose. I did the things I knew from experience had worked before in my periodic efforts to diet. I avoided the empty calories—processed breads, white potatoes, pasta, sweets and sugars—and made the portions of the food I ate about two-thirds smaller. I also increased the intensity of my exercise routine, although I had always exercised. As an airline pilot, I had to stay fit in order to pass my twice-a-year FAA flight physicals.

This is not a "diet" book written by a doctor or a nutritional scientist trying to sell books, diet foods, and/or membership in a weight-loss club. There are plenty of those, some better than others. Any "diet" that reduces what you eat will allow you to lose weight, but that doesn't make the diet healthy or the weight loss sustainable if you feel deprived of the pleasures of good food and drink. I used the word diet in the title of the book in the sense of its Greek origin, the word *diaeta,* which means "manner of living," not in the sense that most Americans think of the word diet as "of eating sparingly," which implies deprivation. I do not feel deprived of anything, including the two martinis I enjoy before dinner. What is meaningful is that I—along with my wife, incidentally—have changed my manner of living.

What follows is about the extremely complex chemistry set that makes up our bodies and the nutrition that we need to be healthy and fueled. This is from my perspective as a layperson. I'm not a nutritional scientist, but I am a quick student and a darn good researcher, and I'd like to share my success with you. There's an advantage to that because, when the scientists dismantle food into its chemical components, it's easy to forget that it is food we're talking about, and if there's something we all really need to know it's how to feed ourselves.

To agribusiness, the factory food industry, and the government agencies, such as the United States Department of Agriculture (USDA) and the Food and Drug Administration (FDA), whose main role is to support them, we are merely a stomach. The more their nutritional scientists can entice us to overfill that stomach with tasty, highly profitable processed foods, usually loaded with cheaply bought empty calories such as high fructose corn syrup (HFCS), (corn is highly subsidized by the federal government), the more money the industry makes. Add to this the financial priority of the medical and drug industries, which is to profit from the treatment of sick people (the majority suffering from chronic illnesses caused by tobacco—also subsidized—obesity, and lack of exercise), and it's no wonder obesity has become an epidemic in the past thirty years.

Nothing in this book should be construed as medical advice—everyone's needs and medical history are different—what's good for me may not be good for you, especially if you're a pregnant woman, child, diabetic, alcoholic, have food allergies, etc. Anyone considering a serious weight loss regimen should do so under the supervision of a doctor, and be checked regularly as I am. Your doctor has to be part of the team. But you're the other half, and you're going to have to really want to live longer and healthier, be willing to change how you live, and learn how to effectively do so in the face of all that's arrayed against you.

L'chaim (to life)!

Chapter 1

WHAT IS A HEALTHY WEIGHT?

Determining a healthy weight is more difficult than it sounds; it varies with each individual's physical needs and height. For instance, someone six-feet-one, at 175 pounds, would be very slim. While someone five-feet-one, carrying 175 pounds would be obese. The medical profession sort of adjusted for the fact that healthy tall people tend to weigh more than shorter people by formulating the Body Mass Index (BMI). You can calculate your BMI mathematically;[1] use the graph on page 7, or on-line calculators, such as the one on the National Institutes of Health: http://www.nhlbisupport.com/bmi/

BMI Categories:	Obesity Class	Risk of chronic disease
Underweight = <18.5		
Normal = 18.5 – 24.9		
Overweight = 25 – 29.9	I	High
Obese = 30 – 39.9	II	Very High
Extremely Obese = 40>	III	Extremely High

Countless studies involving large groups of people have shown that BMIs above 25 increase the risk of dying early, mainly from heart disease and cancer, and should be considered overweight. BMIs of over 30 are considered obese—the higher the number, the higher the risk of chronic disease.

While BMI has proven very useful in determining a healthy weight for men and women ages 19 to 70, it should not be used for competitive athletes and body builders (those whose BMI is high due to great muscle mass), and/or women who are pregnant and/or lactating. Nor is the BMI index to be used for growing children or the elderly who are both frail and sedentary.

Men and women who exercise ten hours a week or more, and athletes, will weigh more because of a higher ratio of lean tissue (muscle, bones, organs) to adipose (fat). For instance, a bodybuilder may have only 8 percent body fat, yet at 250 pounds be considered overweight by the BMI index. Athletes have different needs depending on the sport, i.e., a linebacker or a sumo wrestler needs to have enough body mass (lean and fat) to generate high forces and avoid injury, and a runner needs muscle and only enough fat to store an energy reserve.

Knowing the percentage of fat is actually a better measure of health and fitness than weight. Measuring weight alone does not give any indication of body composition. Excess body fat increases the risk of many diseases, including type 2 diabetes, hypertension, cardiovascular disease and some cancers. In fact, Webster's definition of *Obesity* is "a condition characterized by excessive body fat."

There are various ways to measure body fat; the most common and cheapest is the use of calipers to measure the thickness of the layer of fat under the skin in various parts of the body—this method is not considered very accurate because it depends on the skills of the tester.

Studies indicate that it does matter if fat has accumulated around your belly. You are at increased risk for health problem if your waist circumference is over 40" for men and 35" for women, as measured around your body at the level of your navel.

The gold standard in measuring the percentage of body fat is to weigh a person underwater (hydrostatically) or to use various X-ray and magnetic resonance imaging (MRI) tests, all mostly only used at research centers and not practical for personal use.

I use and recommend a Body Composition Analyzer sold by Tanita. This is an extremely accurate scale and a body fat/BMI analyzer. If you enter your gender, select if you are athletic, enter your age and your height, it will display your weight and either your percentage of body fat or BMI, whichever is selected. It does so by measuring the bioelectrical impedance of your body using a low DC current that measures the percentage of body water—muscle contains a greater percentage of water than fat—and, using scientific logarithms, computes it. (Not to be used by someone on a pacemaker; it may stop your clock.) You can buy a Tanita body fat analyzer for under a couple of hundred dollars; some gyms and sports clubs have them. As a data guy, I feel accurate information is important and I weigh and analyze myself every morning, at the same time. In that way I catch small changes very early and adjust accordingly. Others say check your weight once a week. That doesn't work for me.

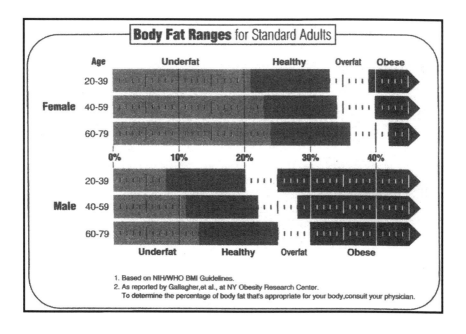

Your ideal weight and fat-lean ratio varies considerably for men and women and by age, but the lowest percentage of body fat considered safe for good health is 5 percent for males and 12 percent for females. The average adult body fat is closer to 15-18 percent for men and 22-25

percent for women. There's little evidence of any benefit when men drop under 8 percent and women drop under 14 percent body fat. We need body fat as an energy reserve, and under the skin and around organs for protection.

How low is too low?

While the average body fat percentage in the United States and Europe is increasing, extremely low body fat percentage is also a health problem. The <u>female athlete triad,</u> which is the combination eating disorders, amenorrhea and osteoporosis attributed to female athletes, highlights the problem; women athletes who lose too much fat risk injury, decreased performance and health issues.

The female athlete triad speaks to three health problems often found in women athletes:

- Low energy availability
- Menstrual disorders
- Weak bones (increased risk of stress fractures and osteoporosis)

An attempt to reduce body fat by extreme measures not only leads to decreased performance, but also can lead to severe health complications. Nutrient deficiencies and fluid/electrolyte imbalance from low food intake can lead to increased risk of fractures, illness, loss of reproductive function, and serious medical conditions such as dehydration, and starvation. The medical complications of this triad involve almost every body function and include the cardiovascular, endocrine, reproductive, skeletal, gastrointestinal, renal, and central nervous systems. About two-thirds of your brain is composed of fats.

My Profile

When I started my weight loss program, I weighed 270 pounds with a 54" waist. At 5'9" (69") my charted BMI was a whopping 40, extremely obese, even though my percentage of body fat didn't exceed 23 percent; you can be overweight or obese with lean muscle mass as well as fat—I was simply much larger than I needed to be; my weight was not an advantage in any way, although in my workouts I could lift heaver weights. Just imagine carrying 100 additional pounds around every moment of every day—each step placing a 270 pound load on the landing leg and foot. As said in the preface, I was suffering from several chronic diseases and I was at extremely high risk for others. I probably didn't develop type 2 diabetes because my percentage of body fat remained within reason.

I'm still 5'9", but with a body weight of 170 lbs and a charted BMI of 25 (on the high side of normal), however, my computed BMI by my body composition analyzer and my percentage of body fat both run between 10 and 12 percent. For my age I'm lean and muscular due to an exercise program that alternates daily routines of 1-hour and an hour and a half (10 hours a week), each day burning about 500 calories; 3,500 calories a week, which is equal to the calories in a pound of fat. (More on the importance of exercise later)

How Do You Rate?

- ◆ Over 60 percent of Americans are overweight.
- ◆ The average woman in the United States is 5'4". If she weighs 152 lbs, her BMI is 26.1, and she's overweight. A healthy weight for a woman of average height would be would be about 134 lbs, unless she's muscular.
- ◆ The average man in the U.S. is 5'9". If he weighs 185 lbs, his BMI is 27.3 – also overweight. A healthy weight for a man of average height would be about 153 lbs, unless he's muscular.

In the Dietary Guidelines for Americans, healthy weights are those corresponding to BMIs between 18.5 and 25, although the risk of heart disease, diabetes, and high blood pressure begins to climb at BMIs of 22 or so. The BMI dietary guideline was formulated by studies that tracked the health of large groups of people. It is the measure used internationally by healthcare professionals and the life insurance industry—you'll learn that quickly enough if you're obese and try to buy life insurance.

Can you be too lean?

Absolutely, malnutrition is a dangerous condition that can cause disease and the breakdown of your body. As omnivores (humans are both plant and meat eaters), we need a wide variety of nutrients, vitamins, and minerals to be healthy. For example, none of the extremely lean, starved prisoners at Auschwitz was healthy. In the same way, smokers may be lean, but few will be in good health for long. Many people smoke for that reason, to be lean, which puts them at extremely high risk for cancer, heart disease, and just about every other ailment that can lay you low. People who are seriously ill tend to lose weight as well—that's the reason why people ask me if I'm okay if they haven't seen me in awhile. And there are some dangerous eating disorders that can be life threatening, such as anorexia nervosa, and bulimia nervosa that mostly afflict young woman. And let's not forget that plenty of people in the world who go to bed hungry.

The bottom line is you need food and drink to live; without it you will die. But what you eat and drink, as well as your BMI and load of body fat, will determine your life expectancy, and exposure to chronic disease (more in the next chapter). The old axiom that you are what you eat is true. Believe it or not, most of the people who are overweight or obese are also undernourished, filling their bodies with calories that do absolutely nothing to support good health—empty calories, are now cheap as dirt, that flood the blood with too much sugar that the body efficiently turns into body fat.

Knowing your body weight and composition is as important to you as annual physical check-ups (which are not covered by most health insurance companies), and periodic breast, prostate, colon, and oral examinations. A healthy body weight—probably what you weighed in college, unless you were overweight—along with not smoking and exercise is your best safeguard against chronic illness, and your best shot at a longer, healthier life.

If you are overweight, don't exercise, smoke, and suffer from chronic disease, a change in your manner of living can mitigate or possibly eliminate your symptoms and potentially give you a longer and healthier life. So it is clear that many of us have a lot of work to do.

Body Mass Index Table

	Normal						Overweight					Obese										Extreme Obesity														
BMI	19	20	21	22	23	24	25	26	27	28	29	30	31	32	33	34	35	36	37	38	39	40	41	42	43	44	45	46	47	48	49	50	51	52	53	54
Height (inches)												Body Weight (pounds)																								
58	91	96	100	105	110	115	119	124	129	134	138	143	148	153	158	162	167	172	177	181	186	191	196	201	205	210	215	220	224	229	234	239	244	248	253	258
59	94	99	104	109	114	119	124	128	133	138	143	148	153	158	163	168	173	178	183	188	193	198	203	208	212	217	222	227	232	237	242	247	252	257	262	267
60	97	102	107	112	118	123	128	133	138	143	148	153	158	163	168	174	179	184	189	194	199	204	209	215	220	225	230	235	240	245	250	255	261	266	271	276
61	100	106	111	116	122	127	132	137	143	148	153	158	164	169	174	180	185	190	195	201	206	211	217	222	227	232	238	243	248	254	259	264	269	275	280	285
62	104	109	115	120	126	131	136	142	147	153	158	164	169	175	180	186	191	196	202	207	213	218	224	229	235	240	246	251	256	262	267	273	278	284	289	295
63	107	113	118	124	130	135	141	146	152	158	163	169	175	180	186	191	197	203	208	214	220	225	231	237	242	248	254	259	265	270	278	282	287	293	299	304
64	110	116	122	128	134	140	145	151	157	163	169	174	180	186	192	197	204	209	215	221	227	232	238	244	250	256	262	267	273	279	285	291	296	302	308	314
65	114	120	126	132	138	144	150	156	162	168	174	180	186	192	198	204	210	216	222	228	234	240	246	252	258	264	270	276	282	288	294	300	306	312	318	324
66	118	124	130	136	142	148	155	161	167	173	179	186	192	198	204	210	216	223	229	235	241	247	253	260	266	272	278	284	291	297	303	309	315	322	328	334
67	121	127	134	140	146	153	159	166	172	178	185	191	198	204	211	217	223	230	236	242	249	255	261	268	274	280	287	293	299	306	312	319	325	331	338	344
68	125	131	138	144	151	158	164	171	177	184	190	197	203	210	216	223	230	236	243	249	256	262	269	276	282	289	295	302	308	315	322	328	335	341	348	354
69	128	135	142	149	155	162	169	176	182	189	196	203	209	216	223	230	236	243	250	257	263	270	277	284	291	297	304	311	318	324	331	338	345	351	358	365
70	132	139	146	153	160	167	174	181	188	195	202	209	216	222	229	236	243	250	257	264	271	278	285	292	299	306	313	320	327	334	341	348	355	362	369	376
71	136	143	150	157	165	172	179	186	193	200	208	215	222	229	236	243	250	257	265	272	279	286	293	301	308	315	322	329	338	343	351	358	365	372	379	386
72	140	147	154	162	169	177	184	191	199	206	213	221	228	235	242	250	258	265	272	279	287	294	302	309	316	324	331	338	346	353	361	368	375	383	390	397
73	144	151	159	166	174	182	189	197	204	212	219	227	235	242	250	257	265	272	280	288	295	302	310	318	325	333	340	348	355	363	371	378	386	393	401	408
74	148	155	163	171	179	186	194	202	210	218	225	233	241	249	256	264	272	280	287	295	303	311	319	326	334	342	350	358	365	373	381	389	396	404	412	420
75	152	160	168	176	184	192	200	208	216	224	232	240	248	256	264	272	279	287	295	303	311	319	327	335	343	351	359	367	375	383	391	399	407	415	423	431
76	156	164	172	180	189	197	205	213	221	230	238	246	254	263	271	279	287	295	304	312	320	328	336	344	353	361	369	377	385	394	402	410	418	426	435	443

Chapter 2

The Obesity Epidemic

One of the volunteer jobs that I enjoy is to serve on the board of directors of the New Hampshire Citizen's Alliance (NHCA), a progressive nonprofit group that advocates for social and economic justice. Following a board meeting (and many compliments about my weight loss), I had the good fortune on the long drive home to tune into an interview with Doctor Richard Carmona, the chairperson of a new group being formed called the Partnership to Fight Chronic Disease (PFCD). Dr. Carmona was the 17th Surgeon General of the United States (2002-2006). He was in New Hampshire to recognize Dr. Susan Lynch, the state's first lady, as chairperson of New Hampshire, joining Ohio, Iowa, and South Carolina. Dr. Lynch is a pediatrician whose specialty is childhood obesity. PFCD's website is http://www. fightchronicdisease.org

I was particularly interested in hearing Dr. Lynch, having campaigned with her and Governor Lynch during my recent unsuccessful run for the state senate. She's an articulate, accomplished woman. NHCA has a long history of advocating for health care and affordable health care-insurance.

What I heard during the next hour absolutely blew me away. I knew I'd had a problem with my health because of being overweight, and had some idea of the problem in the U.S., but I had absolutely no idea of the magnitude of the healthcare crisis it is. Here's how Dr. Carmona layed it out—from the website:

> Chronic diseases, such as asthma, cancer, diabetes, and heart disease, are the leading causes of death and disability in the United States and account for the vast majority of healthcare spending. They affect the quality of life for 133 million Americans and are responsible for seven out of every ten deaths in the U.S.—killing more than 1.7 million Americans a year.

> Chronic diseases are also the primary driver of healthcare costs, accounting for more than 75 cents of every dollar we spend on health issues in this country, as reported by the Centers for Disease Control (CDC). In 2005, this amounted to $1.5 trillion of the $2 trillion spent on healthcare.

> Despite these widespread problems, the issue of chronic disease does not register with large segments of the public and policymakers as an issue of primary concern.

The dollars spent didn't surprise me, I wrote an in depth chapter on the cost of the health care in the United States in my book, *Facing Fascism; The Threat to American Democracy in the 20th Century*. What startled me, however, is that CDC estimates that eliminating three risk factors – **poor diet, inactivity, and smoking** - would prevent:

- 80 percent of heart disease and stroke
- 80 percent of type 2 diabetes
- 40 percent of cancer

Wow! Check the following data at both the PFCD and the Centers for Disease Control (CDC) website: http://www.cdc.gov/nccdphp/dnpa/index.htm

Obesity

The latest data from the Centers for Disease Control (CDC) show more than 30 percent of U.S. adults of 20 years and older

— more than 60 million people — are obese. People with a body Mass Index (BMI) over 30 have an increased risk of developing chronic disease including:

+ Hypertension
+ Dyslipidemia (for example, high total cholesterol or high levels of triglycerides)
+ Type 2 diabetes
+ Coronary heart disease
+ Stroke
+ Gallbladder disease
+ Osteoarthritis
+ Sleep apnea and respiratory problems
+ Some cancers (endometrial, breast, and colon)

Health risks related to obesity can be reduced through proper nutrition and physical activity. However, many Americans are not following a healthy diet. The American Cancer Society reports that more than three-quarters (76.8 percent) of adults eat less than five servings of fruits and vegetables a day.

Many Americans are also not active. CDC research indicates that the direct medical costs associated with physical inactivity totaled nearly $76.6 billion in 2000, and studies show that almost a quarter of Americans do not participate in ANY physical activities.

Smoking

Smoking adversely affects nearly every organ in the body. Research shows that while smoking often leads to various types of cancers, smokers also are at risk of developing cardiovascular disease, respiratory illness and other health problems.

Childhood Obesity

The CDC reports that data from two National Health and Nutrition Examination Survey's (1976-1980, and 2003-2004) show increases in overweight among children and teens. For children aged 2-5 years, the prevalence of overweight increased from 5.0 percent to 13.9 percent; for those aged 6-11years, prevalence increased from 6.5 percent to 18.8 percent; and for those aged 12-19 years, prevalence increased from 5.0 percent to 17.4 percent.

Without change the future is grim.

The Rand Corporation reported in 2000: about 133 million Americans – 45 percent have at least one chronic disease.

The American Diabetes Association estimates that one of three of today's first graders will develop diabetes over the course of their lifetime.

According to the CDC:
In all chronic diseases now account for one-third of the years of potential life lost before age 65.

The number of people diagnosed with diabetes almost doubled from 1995 (4.4 percent) to 2005 (7.3 percent)—there's no reason to believe that number will not continue to escalate.

PFCD:
"Because of increasing rates of obesity…we may see the first generation that will…have shorter life expectancy than their parents."

Former Surgeon General, Richard H. Carmona

National Coalition on Health Care:
- In 2007, health care spending in the United States reached $2.3 trillion, and was projected to reach $3 trillion in 2011. Health care spending is projected to reach $4.2 trillion by 2016.
- Health care spending is 4.3 times the amount spent on defense.
- In 2005, the United States spent 16 percent of its gross domestic product (GDP) on health care. It is projected that the percentage will reach 20 percent by 2016.

- Health care spending accounted for 10.9 percent of the GDP in Switzerland, 10.7 percent in Germany, 9.7 percent in Canada, and 9.5 percent in France, according to the Organization for Economic Cooperation and Development.

The cost of health care and health care insurance is a crisis in the United States and a top issue in 2008 presidential campaign. Forty-six million Americans (over 15 percent) have no health insurance, and many that do are underinsured. Medical bills have become one of the leading reasons for personal bankruptcies. Yet, despite the debates on insurance reform, be it a single-payer governmental system or increased availability of private health insurance, not a word is heard about the driving force behind the skyrocketing cost of healthcare: obesity, lack of exercise and smoking. For these reasons, I'm proud to say, the New Hampshire Citizens Alliance has joined the Partnership to Fight Chronic Diseases—it needs to be out in front as a platform issue for candidates.

When the NHCA board decided to become a partner within PFCD, one of our reservations was that we wouldn't lend our support to any effort that would penalize people for personal poor choices in lifestyle—after all, no one forces a person to eat irresponsibly, to smoke, or not to exercise—the far right characteristically would deny them benefits. As it is, if you're a smoker you can be denied health care and life insurance or be put in a high risk, expensive pool. Yet despite personal choices, no one actually chooses to have a chronic illness; and those that acquire them have been victimized by public policy makers, the healthcare system, the insurance industry, agribusiness, the factory food industry, the tobacco industry, and the media—all of which profit either by stuffing unhealthy food down our throats, smoke into our lungs, or treating illness. Very little is spent on preventive medicine or educating people, especially our children, as to how to eat properly, the importance of exercise, and not poisoning our bodies by smoking. Instead we spend more than $7,000 per person, per year, on the treatment of chronic diseases, 80 percent of which can be avoided.

"We spend, as a society, less than $10 per person, per year, on prevention. We spend more than that on oil changes on our cars…we have got to change the way we do business. We need a better balance in our health care system between prevention and repair work."

Dr. James S. Marks, the U.S. Centers for
Disease Control and Prevention.

Before 2004, Medicare did not consider obesity to be a disease or illness and made no payments for any service in connection with it. The revised 2004 Medicare policy, according Department of Health and Human Services (HHS), "would remove barriers to covering anti-obesity interventions if scientific and medical evidence demonstrates their effectiveness in improving Medicare beneficiaries' health outcomes." Subsequently, Medicare approves some gastric bypass surgery when used for the treatment of diseases caused by obesity, e.g., type 2 diabetes, cardiovascular disease, etc. It was an improvement that offers only drastic surgical intervention after a person is morbidly obese; there are no benefits provided for prevention. (Federal Medicare coverage is only available to people over age 65.)

State-based Medicaid and all but a few private plans pay nothing toward prevention of obesity or for gastric bypass surgery, only to directly treat the various illnesses bought on by obesity.

Obesity in the World
<u>According to the World Health Organization (WHO)</u>
- Globally, there are more than 1 billion overweight adults, at least 300 million of them obese.
- Obesity and overweight pose a major risk for chronic diseases, including type 2 diabetes, cardiovascular disease, hypertension and stroke, and certain forms of cancer.
- The key causes are increased consumption of energy-dense foods high in carbohydrates, and reduced physical activity.

On January 16, 2004, the Bush administration challenged a WHO report that urged nations to take steps to reduce obesity. The WHO recommends eating more fruits and vegetables and limiting fats and salt. It also suggested that governments limit food advertising aimed at children and encourage their citizens to eat healthier foods.

Health and Human Services official William Steiger, questioning the report's findings, said they were based on faulty science. He went on to say in his letter that the report did not adequately address an individual's responsibility to balance one's diet with one's physical activities, and objected to singling out specific types of foods, such as those high in fat and sugar.

"The U.S. government favors dietary guidance that focuses on the total diet, promotes the view that all foods can be part of a healthy and balanced diet, and supports personal responsibility to choose a diet conductive to individual energy balance, weight control and health," wrote Steiger. The dietary guidance that he speaks of is the USDA Food Guidance Pyramid that came out in 1992. Although attacked by scores of studies over the next thirteen years, the pyramid wasn't changed until 2005; it is now called MyPyramid.gov—an interactive website only available on the Internet. The website has few words, lots of color, and paltry advice, obviously largely shaped by the food industries lobby. You can bet that our political leaders are not going to allow the USDA or HHS to cross swords with either the agribusiness or the health-care sector when trillions of dollars are dependent on feeding people junk, and then treating their illnesses. (More on the MyPyramid and other diets later)

> Opensecrets.org reports that between 1998-2007 K Street agribusiness lobbyists spent over $914 million and health-care sector lobbyists over $2.7 billion—that's a lot horsepower.

That was an incredible statement for a HHS official to make considering the obesity epidemic in the U.S.—one that we are exporting to the rest of world with our fast-food chains, our "western diet," giant portions, and unhealthy lifestyle. Because of cheap subsidized farm products in the U.S., agribusiness and food factories can afford to successfully stuff us with highly processed foods that are loaded with salt, trans fats and saturated fats, and unneeded carbohydrates. A must read in this regard is, The *Omnivore's Dilemma,* by Michael Pollan. (Much more on the Western diet later)

Clearly the World Health Organization (U.N.) was on target in suggesting that governments should limit food advertising aimed at children and they should encourage their citizens to eat healthier foods. Instead, the food industry spends countless millions encouraging us to eat what should be called industrial waste! If that's capitalism, and profit alone rules in America, our days are numbered.

Steiger, his bosses at HHS and the USDA, know the data; many Americans aren't choosing a healthy diet and they are getting sick and dying because our government is not protecting them from predatory business practices. Even our schools are not teaching us how to eat defensively, and not to eat all day long, wrong or not. But it can't all be blamed on the Bush administration and laissez-faire far-right economics. Democrats share the responsibility by voting for subsidies that reward farmers for overproducing crops. Instead of being stored in silos, sold overseas, or not grown at all in order to rotate crops, these overproduced crops are broken down in factories into their chemical components, and then reformulated into the highly profitable processed foods that are turning Americans into walking storage units of high energy calories – fat. (More on the food chain in the next chapter)

I'm not suggesting that we return to the dust bowl days before FDR and farm price supports came into play over 60 years ago—rather that we have price supports that encourage the production of quality foods that promote good health on farms that provide good jobs and a sustainable environment. In fact, small farmers benefit very little from farm subsidies compared to large agribusinesses.

The data speaks for itself. The following is a portion of a Factsheet by the Center for Sustainable Systems (University of Michigan): (Enclosed comments are mine.)

Agricultural Production

- ◆ 8% of all farms account for about 68% of agricultural production.
- ◆ A mere 19 cents of every dollar spent on food in 2000 went back to the farm – in1975 it was 40 cents.

- In 2001 – 2002, 53% of the hired crop labor force lacked authorization to work in the United States.
- The rate of groundwater withdrawal exceeds recharge rates in major agricultural regions.
- As a result of nutrient runoff in the agricultural upper regions of the Mississippi River, the average size of the hypoxic "dead zone" in the Gulf of Mexico was over 5,300 sq mi from 2000 to 2005.
- In 2003, 1.8 billion tons of topsoil was lost to erosion – or 200,000 tons a day.
- Despite tenfold increase in insecticide use since 1945, crop lose due to insect damage have nearly doubled.
- Agricultural activities were responsible for 7% of total U.S. greenhouse gas emissions in 2005. Livestock are major contributors.

Consumption Patterns

- In 2000, the U.S. food supply provided 3,800 calories per person per day (nearly double what the average person needs). Accounting for waste, the average American consumed 2,700 calories per day – an increase of 24.5% from 1970. (500 calories a day more than burned will result in a weight gain of about a pound a week.)
- In 2005, Americans ate 200 pounds of meat per person, which is up 22 pounds from 1970. Over half the grains grown are fed to animals.
- The average American eats 32 teaspoons of caloric sweeteners – mostly sucrose and corn sweeteners (HFCS) – per day!
- In 2004, 66% of U.S. adults were either overweight or obese, defined as having a body mass index of 25 or more.
- Poor nutrition and physical inactivity accounted for 400,000 premature deaths in 2000, Diet contributes to heart disease, certain cancer, and stroke – the three major causes of U.S. deaths.

Smoking

Before moving on, a few words about smoking. Simply, you can't eat healthy and be healthy if you smoke—it's pointedly foolish to think that you can.

The problem is that nicotine is addictive and readily available to any adult in the United States and throughout the world. All the tobacco industry has to do is get you hooked and you're theirs.

When the FAA banned smoking on domestic and international flights, airlines, including mine, were forced to run seminars for captains whose responsibility it was to enforce the regulations. It wasn't too bad on shorter flights, but on long flights, some over ten hours, we'd have smokers literally bouncing off the walls, or, more dangerously, smoking in the lavatories, setting off smoke detectors, and, worse, putting smoldering butts in the trash. The focus was to avoid having passengers removed from the aircraft and incarcerated by having the pilot and crew understand the severity of the addiction, not to condone the behavior.

As this is written, I have a 43-year-old daughter-in-law who is seriously ill with a form of lung disease brought about by smoking. She's tried repeatedly to kick the habit but couldn't do it. Nor does the family have health insurance that would help her to kick the habit—our insurers, it seems, would rather pay to treat the illness.

My father died from a combination of cancers of the larynx and lymphoma, and cardiovascular disease that began to take him down at age 62 and killed him within ten years of pain and struggle. He was a two-pack-a-day smoker. He would light up in the morning when his feet hit the ground—as a child the smoke would wake me up. Six of his siblings, all heavy smokers, also died young.

Those of us who are senior citizens all have known countless people who have suffered and died from various cancers, emphysema, or cardiovascular disease because of smoking; it's a national, if not worldwide tragedy. The trouble is children don't have that life experience, and in their youth can't imagine getting terribly ill in middle age and having their life cut short. Although cigarettes can legally be sold only to adults, teenagers have no trouble getting them; just go by any high school.

The question is why are cigarettes legal when narcotics and other dangerous drugs are not? Smoking advocates will say the packs are labeled as being dangerous to your health—it should be a matter of personal responsibility. Alcohol, also, can be dangerous and addictive. We tried prohibition and look what happened to that. The answer is that, used responsibly and in moderation, alcohol does not hurt most people, smoking does. There is no way to smoke responsibly.

Of course the United States is not alone in allowing the legal sale of cigarettes to adults; just about every country does. The reason is simple. Governments, certainly our own state and federal governments tax the hell out of cigarettes—they're partners with the tobacco industry. My state of New Hampshire purposefully keeps its cigarette tax substantially lower than its border states to encourage people to shop for them at our border stores. How much of that revenue is put into the healthcare system to treat the diseases caused by cigarettes, and into the school system to educate our children about the terrible results of smoking? Zero; all the money goes into the general fund.

As Yul Brynner put it in a recorded television message broadcast after his death from lung cancer on October 10, 1985, "Now that I'm gone, I tell you, don't smoke." Brynner, like most actors of his day, characteristically smoked on screen and off.

It's my advice too. I've never smoked (though I got gassed with second-hand smoke for about twenty-five years on airliners) so I can't claim to have had the will power to stop. To beat it you have to really deep in your heart realize it's a matter of your life or your death. I suggest that if you think you don't have the will power to do so you visit almost any major hospital and find a patient dying of lung cancer or emphysema, watch them choking and gasping for enough breath that will never come again. I think videos of them should be part of all high school curriculums.

Chapter 3

Eaters and Food

If you're going to survive in today's world and not get fattened up like cattle at a Concentrated Animal Feeding Operation (CAFO), you're going to have to know some basic stuff about food in order to make wise eating decisions. Today's giant supermarkets are every bit as dangerous as the primitive world early humans lived in hundreds of thousands of years ago as hunter-gathers.

We and other critters large and small can be lumped into three categories of eaters, although there are plenty of crossovers—some forced by agribusiness—herbivores (strict vegetarians), carnivores (strict meat-eaters), and omnivores (those that opportunistically eat both meat and plants). Carnivores generally eat herbivores, but can eat omnivores, and sometimes other carnivores. A few examples of mammals in each category:

Herbivores

Many of the plants that grow on earth cannot be used directly by humans as food; we do not have the multiple stomachs needed (which act like fermenting vats) to digest grasses or vegetation; ruminants do. Ruminants include cattle, buffalo, sheep, goats, deer, elk, giraffes and camels. Other plant eaters include horses, rhinos, and colobine monkeys; these have posterior, hindgut sacks to accomplish digestion.

Herbivores also have teeth adapted to chewing plants, with big molars designed to help them grind up leaves, seeds and twigs.

Carnivores

Carnivores are predators. They hunt and eat other animals to survive, which requires the tremendous amount of food energy that they get from the energy-dense meat they eat. Their jaws are large and powerful with sharp teeth adapted for ripping meat and sharp claws that help them catch prey. Carnivores include lions, tigers, bobcats, leopards, polar bears, wolves and coyotes.

Omnivores

Omnivores are animals that eat both plants and animals as their primary food. Humans are omnivores. We're opportunistic, general feeders not adapted to eat and digest either meat or plant material exclusively. Most omnivores are not cannibalistic, although humans have recorded instances of having eaten others to survive, and some primitive tribes have practiced cannibalism—there seems to be a biological reason why animals don't eat their own species. For instance, feeding beef products to fatten beef at CAFOs is thought to cause bovine spongiform encephalopathy (BSE), commonly known as mad-cow disease—the practice is outlawed in the United States and all other advanced countries. Omnivores include humans, pigs, most bears, skunks, most rodents, and domestic dogs and cats. Our two Airedales and Bengal cats definitely prefer meat to kibble or vegetables—they're sort of reluctant omnivores, but they have the ability to digest both.

Early Man

Just imagine how difficult it was for early man to survive; he was both the predator and the prey. The various offshoots of early man, which date back about three-and-half million years, also had very small brains with which to work it out—about a third of the size of modern man. Because modern man is physically larger, the growth of brains as a percentage of body mass only doubled from about 1 percent to 2 percent. It's interesting to note that our brains today at 2 percent of body mass consume a full 20 percent of our food energy, mainly in the form glucose (blood sugar that can be used by cells)—it's one of the reasons why it's so easy for the food industry to shove sugars (particularly cheap HFCS) down our throats. Our brains love it.

In keeping with Darwin's theory of the survival of the fittest, only those early humans that developed larger brains were able to beat the odds and survive. The big change in brain size and intelligence only began to occur about 200,000 years ago. This, scientists believe, was linked to the availability of fats, particularly the essential families of omega 3, and omega 6 fatty acids. About two-thirds of your brain is composed of fat—so, without offense, we're all fat heads.

By analyzing the bones of Neanderthals who lived 28,000 to 130,000 years ago in Europe, scientists have determined that they ate lots of red meat from the larger animals that roamed the continent at the time; they had some omega 6 and omega 3 from flowering seed plants but not in abundance. In contrast, the bones of early man that lived near water indicate they ate seafoods, like shellfish, that could be collected easily. These ancestors with a diet rich in omega 3 fatty acids combined with a supply of omega 6 fatty acids in their diet, developed larger, more intelligent brains. As a result, inland early men got stuck at a brain capacity not much greater than that of a chimpanzee and became extinct.

As early man got more intelligent he was able to develop stone tools (about 150,000 years ago) that could ignite fires—rather than trying in vain to keep one burning after a lightning strike, which supposedly they did. Fire enabled cooking, which gave them the ability to soften foods that couldn't be digested before, and fire, which helped keep predators away. As a result man's food choices were expanded and the species survived to be the modern man we are today.

All of which begs the question, how do humans then and now distinguish between what's edible and what's harmful to eat? Nature has given us certain sensual safeguards. We're attracted to good smells, good taste, pleasing texture, and colors that get our attention, and repelled by others like decay (death and rotten things), things that taste bad, hurt the mouth, and by feces. Unfortunately, today's nutritional scientists can chemically create great tastes, smells, and textures in food products that should have skull and crossbones on the label. In eating them, Americans are growing fatter, and less healthy—fortunately, we no longer have saber-tooth tigers chasing after us or tasty morsels we'd be.

The next great breakthrough in our family tree was probably farming and raising animals for food. This probably first occurred between ten of twelve thousand years ago in the Nile Valley and Mesopotamia. Basic human progress ever since has largely been measured in man's ability to raise, store and preserve food, protect property, and thus ward off starvation. In today's modern world this equates to protecting natural resources, like oil, natural gas, coal, water, and protecting food supplies, industry, and capital markets; it is still basically all about food, shelter, and survival.

Famine and Starvation

Total starvation, the deprivation of food and water, results in death within 10-12 days; if water alone is taken, a person may survive up to 40 days. Without water, the human body becomes dehydrated very quickly.

In cases of famine, when water but very little food is available, death usually results from diseases such as typhus, tuberculosis, anemia, or pneumonia, because the lack of protein compromises the body's ability to rebuild itself and build the antibodies to fight the disease.

Famine and starvation have plagued mankind throughout history, and still do today in countries like Darfur, Somalia, and Eritrea. The descendents of Irish immigrants still speak of the Potato Famine of the 1840s that their ancestors fled. That famine took an estimated one million lives, and drove another two million to travel to the Continent or to the United States.

As this is written, there's great concern that the number of Americans receiving food stamps is projected to reach 28 million in 2009, the highest level since the aid program began in the 1960s. To qualify, recipients must have near-poverty incomes to receive benefits that average $100 a month per family member—pathetic generosity for the richest nation on earth. America's food pantries and the World Food Bank are also under tremendous strain. It's a sad dichotomy that while so many of us are suffering from obesity, and the chronic illnesses it heralds, others in the world are starving.

Eat to Live, Not Live to Eat

In modern recorded history opulent, fat people, have always existed, but obesity has only become a national and world epidemic in the last thirty years or so. In fact, up until the twentieth century most people thought that being stout was a sign of affluence, and that plenty of flesh on the bone helped fight disease and was healthy. If you look at renaissance art you see voluptuous women, not slender chicks. We now know that being round is not healthy, and most people think of it as slothful.

In the last chapter I placed a lot of responsibility for obesity on agribusiness, the food factories, the United States Department of Agriculture, and the Department of Health and Human Services—more about them and the role the American Heart Association later in the book. The important thing is that every person, including children, as they're old enough to understand, has to take responsibility for their own health, eat properly, and attain and keep a healthy weight.

Chapter 4
Calories and Metabolism

The old adage that you are what you eat happens to be true. Chemically, humans, just like the dinosaurs, other animals, and plants, are a carbon life form; as such, both animal and plant fats can and are used to produce bio-diesel fuel, and just about anything that grows, particularly corn and sugar beets is used to produce ethanol. In the past surplus corn was used to make Bourbon whisky. Now the price of corn is at an all-time high because it is being used to produce ethanol for our cars. With the price of oil well over $140 a barrel (July 2008), it is jacking up the price of food. Corn is used for animal feed, and agriculture uses a tremendous amount of oil and natural gas both to run farm equipment, deliver products, and in the process of producing nitrogen fertilizers. It's a double whammy. (More latter)

All of our food energy comes, at its origin, from the sun. Plants need sunlight for the process of photosynthesis to grow; animal eat the plants; we eat both the plants and the animals that eat the plants—works out pretty well. It's hard to believe that other planets circling other stars in the universe would not also have the elements to sustain life, but so far planet Earth is the only one we knows of, so we had better take good care of her.

Most of the human body is made up of water, H_2O, with cells consisting of 65-90% water by weight. It therefore isn't surprising that most of the human body is oxygen. Carbon, the basic unit for organic molecules, comes in second. 99% of the mass of the human body is made up of just six elements: oxygen, carbon, hydrogen, calcium, and phosphorus.

1. Oxygen (65%)
2. Carbon (18%)
3. Hydrogen (10%)
4. Nitrogen (3%)
5. Calcium (1.5%)
6. Phosphorus (1.0%)
7. Potassium (0.35%)
8. Sulfur (0.25%)
9. Sodium (0.15%)
10. Magnesium (0.05%)
11. Copper, Zinc, Selenium, Molybdenum, Fluorine, Chlorine, Iodine, Manganese, Cobalt, Iron (0.70%)
12. Lithium, Strontium, Aluminum, Silicon, Lead, Vanadium, Arsenic, Bromine (trace amounts)

Reference: H.A. Harper, V.

W. Rodwell, P.A. Mayes, *Review of Physiological Chemistry*, 16th ed., Lange Medical Publications, Los altos, California 1977.

Food provides the energy for your body, and the nutrients that allow your body to grow, regenerate, and repair. Getting to know which nutrients are in which foods, and how much food-energy those nutrients have, will help you understand something of the complex relationship between your food and your body, and help you maintain a healthy weight.

The amount of energy a particular food can deliver is measured in calories. A food calorie is the amount of heat needed to raise the temperature of a liter of water (just over a quart) from 14.5^0C to 15.5^0C. As a reference point, a food calorie is the amount energy a 165-pound person burns each minute at rest.

Calories in Micronutrients

Fat: 1 gram = 9 calories

Protein: 1 gram = 4 calories

Carbohydrates: 1 gram = 4 calories

Biologically, a human adult is built out of approximately 100 trillion cells (10^{14}), larger people more cells, smaller ones less. In the nine months from conception to birth, just one cell, or zygote, will divide and differentiate into all the cells that comprise all the different components of the human body—all built from nutrients eaten by the mother and passed on to the fetus. Every 3 – 6 months after birth (until death) 98 percent of your atoms will be replaced from your environment, mostly in the form of food. On a cellular basis, a child will grow into adulthood by the division and addition of cells; some cells die and are replaced, and as the child grows others are added.

As an adult, the process of cell replacement, addition, or subtraction is continued until we die. Consequently, whatever your age, your body is many years younger. In fact, if you are middle aged, most of your cells may be just 10 years old or less. Although we think of our body as a fairly permanent structure, most of it is in a constant state of flux as old cells are discarded and new ones generate in their place. The turnover time depends in part on the workload endured by the cells.

The cells lining the stomach really have a tough time and last only five days; red blood cells, after traveling nearly 1,000 miles through the circulatory system, last about 120 days. And so the list of tissue goes: The epidermis, or surface layer of the skin, about two weeks, an adult liver between 300 to 500 days. Other tissues have lifetimes measured in years, not days, but are still far from permanent. Even the bones have a nonstop makeover—the adult human skeleton is thought to be replaced every ten years or so.

The only pieces of the body that seem to last a lifetime are the neurons of the cerebral cortex, the inner lens cells of the eye and perhaps the muscle cells of the heart.

The obvious question is if we're constantly rebuilding ourselves, why do we die—the oldest reported human was about 120 years of age. Some experts think the root cause is that the DNA accumulates mutations and its information is gradually degraded. Others blame the DNA of the mitochondria, which lack the repair mechanisms available for the chromosomes. A third theory is that the stem cells that are the source of new cells in each tissue eventually grow feeble with age.

The bad news about fat cells is that the body can always make more of them, and compared with other cells they are extremely long-lived. A lean adult has about 40 billion fat cells, an obese one at least two to three times that. And obese people have much larger fat cells than lean ones. If a person keeps overeating, fat cells will grow and grow, looking as if they are about to pop. When they reach the limit, they don't divide; they send a signal to nearby immature cells to start dividing to produce more fat cells.

Mitochondria

Mitochondria are spherical or rod-shaped organelles found within cells. They are regarded as the "powerhouse of the cell" because they are capable of using glucose and oxygen to produce energy for use in many metabolic processes. Therefore, it is not surprising to find several mitochondria in high energy-requiring cells, such as brain and muscle cells.

Metabolism

Metabolism is the chemical processes by which your body converts food into energy while other substances, necessary for life, are synthesized. During this complex biochemical process, calories—from carbohydrates, fats, proteins, and alcohol—are combined with oxygen within cells by the mitochondria to release the energy your body needs to function.

Even at rest your body requires quite a lot of energy for the basics, such as, maintaining body temperature (normal is 37° C – 98.6° F), circulating blood (about 2,000 gal. a day), breathing, adjusting hormone levels, and growing and repairing cells. Calories burned to cover these basic functions are your basal metabolic rate (BMR). For most people BMR is the largest portion of energy use, about two-thirds to three-quarters of the calories burned each day. BMR stays fairly constant and isn't easily changed.

The basal metabolic rate (BMR) for an average 165-pound person is about 1,440 calories. But many factors influence caloric requirements, body size and composition, age, and sex.

- Body size and composition. Obviously a bigger body mass requires more energy (calories) than a smaller one. But, referring back to chapter 1, your body's composition is a big factor. Muscle burns more calories than fat, even at rest. So the more muscle you have in relation to fat, the higher your basal metabolic rate. You need to know that ratio. I measure mine daily on a Tanita body composition analyzer—my percentage of body fat runs between 10 percent and 12 percent, which is excellent for a man 71 years of age.

- Age. As you grow older, the amount of muscle tends to decrease and fat accounts for more of your weight. Metabolism also slows naturally with age. You have a choice to avoid gaining weight; either reduce your caloric intake, or increase your physical activity.

- Sex. Men usually have less body fat and more muscle than women of the same age and weight. For this reason men generally have a higher basal metabolism rate and burn more calories than women do.

As men age, muscle mass can also decline owing to decreased production of sex (testosterone) and growth hormones—a sort of male menopause. Because of my symptoms, I was tested (a simple blood test) and found to have an extremely low testosterone level. My doctor prescribed a testosterone supplement called AndroGel, which is applied topically once a day. This is not the "doping" that athletes illegally use by any stretch of the imagination. Simply increasing my hormone level to the normal range made a world of difference for me, and I believe the deficiency was one of the reasons for my weight gain. I also believe the condition is largely under-diagnosed, and the symptoms disregarded as normal with aging. They are not normal.

Your total energy expenditure or the number of calories your body burns each day is the sum of the following factors: basal metabolic rate

(BMR); calories used in food processing, which is about 10 percent of calories used each day; and calories burned by physical activity.

Physical activity—any movement, whether it's walking up the stairs and not taking the elevator, walking instead of driving, playing tennis, lifting weights, or using a treadmill or rowing machine accounts for the remainder of the calories used. You control the number of calories burned depending on the frequency, duration and intensity of your activities. I personally try to be physically active in the everyday things I do, and I exercise between one and one-an-half hours just about every day at a moderate to high intensity. The exercise alone is worth about 500 calories a day, 3,500 calories a week, or about a pound of fat.

All of us have known people who seem to be able to eat anything and never gain an ounce, and others who say they can't shed a pound because they have "low metabolism." Sorry guys, weight is rarely linked to inherited metabolism; instead, it's the old formula: calories consumed versus calories burned—take in fewer calories, and/or increase your physical activity and you lose weight. That said, if you lose muscle mass due to aging and lack of physical activity you will decreased your BMR and have to eat less or you will gain weight. (See Chapter 15)

Chapter 5

The Components of Food

In the last chapter we talked about food energy (calories), and how the body uses that energy through metabolism. Now we'll move on to the other half of what food is—nutrients, or the chemical building blocks that allow the body to grow, regenerate, and repair. We'll also learn why eating these nutrients carelessly can shorten your life and kill you.

In the 19th century, chemists and physiologists studying the composition of foods and the nutritional requirements of humans and animals found that diets needed to include the complex nitrogenous compounds called "proteins" that, with water, form the bulk of our lean tissues. Together with fats, and carbohydrates (starch and sugars) that all provide useable energy during oxidation in the body. These foods, proteins, carbohydrates, and fats, are classified as macronutrients or the nutrients that the body uses in large amounts.

These scientist also knew that bones contain high concentrations of lime (calcium oxide) and phosphate salts and that the body, generally, has a variety of other mineral salts, though it was felt that mixed diets normally supplied adequate quantities of all these without any need for special precautions.

As time would tell, the early scientists were both right and wrong; deficiency in the diet of essential micronutrients (nutritional components such as vitamins that are present in very small amounts) were then the unknown cause of prevalent diseases such as, scurvy (vitamin C, ascorbic acid), beriberi (vitamin B1, thiamin), and pellagra (B3, niacin). Vitamins (carbon-containing compounds) were originally discovered by studying the deficiency in the diets that caused the diseases—in the diseases listed above, the vitamin deficiencies are shown in parentheses. A total of thirteen vitamins are now known. And more and more it looks like cancer, heart disease, stroke, diabetes, osteoporosis, and other chronic diseases are in part either diseases of food deficiency, food overload, or both.

Most scientists agree that what we know today about phytonutrients (components from plants that have health benefits) is just the tip of the iceberg. Consequently, it behooves us to be very careful about accepting the foods being produced by giant commercial farms and concentrated animal feeding operations (CAFOs) as either safe or adequate. We may not be getting all the natural nutrients we need from nutrient depleted soils, and may be eating insecticides, hormones, and antibiotics that are harmful to our health. This is increasingly problematic because generations of Americans now think that food originates at the supermarket. Our connection to the farm and its plants, fruits, and animals is no longer obvious to many, which marks us easy prey for those whose main interest is the bottom line, not our health. Politicians know, before even giving consideration to legislating laws that would increase the quality of food, that in these economically hard times keeping the price of food down is far more important to most of their constituents. In essence quantity and low prices trump quality. All this is set against a backdrop of a looming world food shortage as countries, including the United States, subsidize the growing of biofuel crops to compete with food crops; and as urbanization and development is using up farmlands, and while China and other emerging nations are demanding more meats and energy-dense foods.

The early scientists did have it right in recognizing that a diet composed of many foods, along with sunlight, and water is healthy—though their choice of which foods to eat and those to avoid would be far different than what's thought of as a healthy diet today. Today's nutritionists also seem to agree that taking a one-a-day vitamin and mineral supplement offers an insurance policy against deficiency, while taking additional antioxidants like vitamins A, C, and E may actually be harmful. Also, people who have precancerous growths or cancer should check with their doctor before taking any vitamin supplement—it may act as a double-edged sword.

Macronutrients

Here we'll begin to concentrate on the macronutrients or major nutritional components that are present in relatively large amounts; these are fat, carbohydrates, and protein. All three have calories as well as nutrients; here are the numbers of calories each has:

Fat:	1 gram = 9 calories
Carbohydrates:	1 gram = 4 calories
Protein:	1 gram = 4 calories

Note that fat has over twice the number of calories per gram than carbohydrates and protein. (FYI: 1 ounce = 28.35 grams, ½ pound = 226.796 grams, 1 pound = 453.592 grams)

Note. The USDA Agricultural Research Service lists the individual nutritional contents of about 1,200 foods, all the macronutrients, micronutrients, vitamins, minerals, and cholesterol; the whole ten yards. The report is titled USDA National Nutrient Database for Standard Reference, Release 20. It can be found at: http://www.ars.usda.gov/Main/docs.htm?docid=15869

Much of the technical information in this book was researched at the Harvard School of Public Health's (HSPH) website and a book titled, *Eat, Drink, and Be Healthy,* The Harvard Medical School Guide To Healthy Eating, by Walter C. Willett, M.D., with Patrick J. Skerrett. Co-Developed with The Harvard School of Public Health. The HSPH website is: http://www.hsph.harvard.edu/nutritionsource/index.html

In my research I've checked all the information used in this book with multiple reliable sources (see Credits), and have found the nutritional information offered by Dr. Willett in his book, and that of the Harvard School of Public Health to be pretty much the gold standard.

The faculty members of the Harvard School of Public Heath also created their own Healthy Eating Pyramid that fixes the fundamental flaws of USDA pyramid. As said, I'm not a nutritional scientist, but I've used most of Healthy Eating Pyramid's recommendations in my personal health program, lost a hundred pounds, and I'm easily maintaining a healthy weight, so I know it works. I think of it as my Italian heritage food—sort of an articulated Mediterranean diet. There are many countries bordering Mediterranean Sea; consequently there is no such thing as one diet for all called The Mediterranean Diet. We'll compare regional diets later.

Fats & Cholesterol

Going back to the early to mid-1950s the growing prevalence of heart disease in America was running up warning flags. Conventional thought was that: 1) Higher levels of fat in the diet increase blood cholesterol levels; and 2) Higher cholesterol levels increase the chances of having a heart attack or developing other forms of cardiovascular disease. Thus it should follow that eating less fat should decrease the rate of heart disease. Referring to this correlation, Dr. Willett wrote the following:

"This simple diet-heart hypothesis leaves a lot out of other factors, that the American Heart Association (AHA) addressed reasonably well in 1957 when, based only on limited data, it set out its first dietary guidelines. Notice they hedged their bets by using the word *may*. They said: 1) Diet may play an important role in the development of heart disease. 2) Both the fat content *and total calories in the diet* (italics added) are probably important. 3) The ratio between saturated fats and unsaturated fats may be the basic determinant, and people should get more unsaturated fats and less saturated fat. 4) A wide variety of other factors besides fat, both dietary and nondietary, may be important."

Unfortunately over the years the American Heart Association, the National Cholesterol Education Program, other influential groups, and finally the USDA with its 1992 Food Guide Pyramid, apparently collectively decided that Americans were too stupid to understand a concept of good-fat/bad-fat. Instead they settled on the simpler "all fat is bad" message.

Consequently, we've all had it drummed into us "eat a low-fat, low cholesterol diet" to lose weight and prevent heart disease, a recommendation that's been a total disaster. In the past 25 years Americans have statistically, unarguably, gotten fatter and fatter. Nor has a low fat diet prevented breast cancer or colon cancer, as has been touted. Detailed research, much of it done at Harvard, shows that the total amount of fat in the diet, whether high or low, isn't linked with disease. What really matters is the type of fat in the diet.

What is becoming evident is that bad fats, meaning saturated and trans-fats increase the risk of certain diseases while good fats, meaning monounsaturated and polyunsaturated fats, lower the risk. The trick is to substitute good fats for bad fats. The latest consensus of advice recommends getting between 20 percent and 35 percent of daily calories from fats, limit saturated fats to 10 percent, and eliminating trans-fats altogether if possible. [10 percent of a 2,000-calorie diet is 200 calories, 22.2 grams or slightly less than 1 ounce; 30 percent is 600 calories, 66.6 grams or slightly less than 3 ounces.]

What happened was that people cut down on fat—both the good and the bad fats—and substituted comfort food carbohydrates such as; white bread, potatoes, pasta, white rice, and inexpensive sodas containing high fructose corn syrup (HFCS). Add to these the many new tasty products that are being manufactured at food factories that contain trans-fats and we've got the result, an obesity epidemic with a tremendous increase of chronic disease. It's a terrible diet that: 1) lowers the good HDL (high-density lipoprotein) while increasing the bad LDL (low-density lipoprotein), producing generations of people at higher risk of developing cardiovascular disease while gobbling expensive cholesterol lowering drugs, and 2) is the key ingredients for adult-onset diabetes, now called type 2 diabetes, which is caused by large spikes of blood sugar (glucose) levels and a constant demand on the pancreas to make insulin that it eventually fails to provide.

But boy, America's so-called "western" diet sure makes money for the pharmaceutical industry; they've never had it so good. In 2002, the top ten Fortune 500 drug companies alone showed a profit of over $35 billion on $217 billion in sales.

In 2005, expenditures for prescription drugs were $200.7 billion, five times the $40.3 billion spent in 1990.

The U.S. Department of Health and Human Services projects national prescription drug spending will increase 148 percent from 2005-2016.

The USDA 2005, Dietary Guidelines for Americans called MyPyramid now does recognize the potential health benefits from monounsaturated and polyunsaturated fats, but in other ways continues to cave in to the food lobbyists and offers poor guidance. (More on MyPyramid and Dueling Diets later)

Chapter 6

Fats

Cholesterol and Heart Disease

The latest scientific thought is that cholesterol in the diet is not nearly the demon it has been made out to be. Cholesterol in the bloodstream is what's most important. High blood cholesterol levels greatly increase the risk of heart disease. Actually you make about 75 percent of blood cholesterol in your liver; only 25 percent is absorbed from food. Consequently, even vegetarians who eat no dietary cholesterol can have high blood cholesterol. That said, the American Heart Association recommends eating less than 300 milligrams of cholesterol a day. Those who have trouble controlling their cholesterol should probably remain cautious; reducing the amount of cholesterol in the diet can have a small but helpful impact on blood cholesterol.

Cholesterol, which is itself not a fat, is a very important part of our body chemistry. It's needed to make cell membranes, and the critical sheaths around nerves, and it's the building block from which the body makes many hormones. What the scientists established in the early 1960s and 70s that prompted the anti-dietary fat pronouncements, was a link between high blood cholesterol levels and heart disease. Deposits of cholesterol called plaque can build inside arteries to restrict or even stop blood flow. Or the plaque can rupture causing a heart attack, stroke, or sudden death.

Your body uses fats as a major energy source for cells, and to make the adipose tissue that stores energy, cushions and protects vital organs, and provides insulation. In order to do this fats must get from the digestive system to your cells, which is problematic since like oil and water, fats and blood don't mix. If your intestines or liver dumped digested fats into your blood, they would congeal into unusable globs. Instead fat is packaged into protein-covered particles that mix easily with blood and flow with it. These tiny particles, called lipoproteins (lipids plus protein), contain some cholesterol to help stabilize the particles.

Your bloodstream carries many sizes and shapes of fat-transporting particles. The balance of fat and protein they contain classifies lipoproteins. Those with a little fat and a lot of protein are heavier and denser than the lighter, fluffier, and less dense particles that have more fat than protein. The proteins also do more than just shield fat from water; they act as address labels that help the body route fat-filled particles to specific destinations.

With regard to heart disease, the most important lipoproteins are high-density lipoproteins (HDL), low-density lipoproteins (LDL), and very-low-density lipoproteins (VLDL), which is composed of triglycerides.

HDL (high-density lipoprotein) cholesterol helps remove fat from the body by binding with it in the blood stream and carrying it back to the liver for disposal. It is sometimes called "good cholesterol." A high level of HDL cholesterol may lower your chances of developing heart disease or stroke.

LDL (low-density lipoprotein) cholesterol carries mostly fat and only a small amount of protein from the liver to other parts of the body. It is sometimes called "bad cholesterol." A high LDL cholesterol level may increase your chances of developing heart disease.

VLDL (very-low-density lipoprotein) cholesterol contains very little protein. The main purpose of VLDL is to distribute the triglyceride produced by your liver. A high VLDL cholesterol level can cause the buildup of cholesterol in your arteries and increase your risk of heart disease and stroke.

Triglycerides are a type if fat the body uses to store energy. Only small amounts are found in the blood. Having a high triglyceride level along with high LDL cholesterol may increase your chances of having heart disease more than having only a high LDL cholesterol level.

For adults 20 years of age or older, the National Cholesterol Education Program recommends the following optimal levels:
- Total cholesterol less than 200 milligrams per deciliter (mg/dl)
- HDL cholesterol levels greater than 40 mg/dl
- LDL cholesterol levels less than 100 mg/dl

For triglycerides:
- Normal   Less than 150 mg/dl
- Borderline-high   150 to 199 mg/dl
- High   200 to 499 mg/dl
- Very high   500 mg/dl or higher

These are based on fasting plasma triglyceride levels.

The Good Fats

Monounsaturated Fat Its main source is olives, olive oil, canola oil, peanut oil, cashews, almonds, peanuts, other nuts, and avocados. The fat at room temperature is a liquid. Its effect on cholesterol levels compared to carbohydrates is to lower LDL and raises HDL.

Polyunsaturated Fat Its main source is corn, soybean, safflower, cottonseed oils, and fish. The fat at room temperature is a liquid. Its effect on cholesterol levels compared to carbohydrates is to lower LDL and raises HDL.

The Bad

Saturated Fat Its main source is red meat, meat products, whole milk, cheese, ice cream, eggs, chocolate, coconuts, coconut milk, and coconut oil. The fat at room temperature is a solid; i.e., you can melt butter but when it cools it returns to a solid. There are about two dozen different saturated fats that exist in nature. Their effect on cholesterol and atherosclerosis (artery-clogging) varies in badness. The saturated fats in butter and other dairy products most strongly increase LDL (bad) cholesterol. Those in beef fat don't increase LDL quite as badly and those in chocolate and cocoa even less. _

The tricky part is all three categories of fat are rarely found alone. For instance, olive oil contains 13 percent saturated fat, 72 percent monounsaturated fat, and 8 percent polyunsaturated fat. Palm oil, which is widely used in some parts of the world, contains 87 percent saturated oil, 6 percent monounsaturated unsaturated fat, and 2 percent polyunsaturated fat.

And so it goes in many foods; a sirloin steak (trimmed) contains 6 percent total fat, 2 percent saturated fat, but also about 2 percent monounsaturated fat, and a trace of polyunsaturated fat—altogether not too bad, plus a lot of protein. By comparison, a fast food double hamburger contains 15 percent total fat, 6 percent saturated fat, 6 percent monounsaturated fat, 0.0 percent polyunsaturated fat—not good at all.

Herring (an oily fish) contains 18 percent total fat, just 2 percent saturated fat, but a whopping 12 percent of monounsaturated fat, and 2 percent polyunsaturated fat, which can be subdivided into essential omega 3 and omega 6 fatty acids. Our bodies can't make polyunsaturated fats; we have to get them from food and fish is an excellent source. So herring and other oily fish are a good fat choice that would be omitted from a low total fat diet.

The Ugly

Trans Fats These are fats that do not appear in nature. They are manufactured by heating liquid polyunsaturated vegetable oils in the presence of hydrogen by a process known as hydrogenation. The more hydrogenated an oil is, the harder it will be at room temperature. For example, a spreadable tub of margarine is less hydrogenated and has less trans fats than stick margarine.

The hydrogenation process and margarine was discovered in WW I for use as butter substitute, and widely used in WW II because of food rationing. I remember it as a kid; you had to squeeze in a tube of yucky artificial yellow coloring.

Most trans-fats are found in commercially baked goods, margarines, snack foods, and processed foods (junk foods). Commercially prepared fried foods, such as French fries and onion rings, contain lots of trans fats. Up until 2008, fast food restaurants like McDonald's used this death glop in just about everything they cooked, even those healthy Chicken McNuggets. They'd still be doing it if it weren't for Mayor Michael Bloomberg and the City of New York. In December 2006, New York City became the first city in the nation to ban artery-clogging artificial trans fats at restaurants. The city gave restaurants until July 1, 2008 to eliminate trans fats from all foods. Philadelphia, Stamford, Conn., and Montgomery County, Md., have done so as well. On July 25, 2008, California became the first state to ban trans fats in restaurants, when Gov. Arnold Schwarzenegger signed a bill to phase out their use. Under the new law, trans fats, must be eliminated from restaurant products beginning in 2010, and from all retail baked goods by 2011. Packaged foods will be exempt. In response some fast food chains have begun to move away from trans fats nationwide, others have not.[2]

Trans fats should be avoided completely; they are deadly and contribute to no less than 600,000 deaths a year due to heart disease. Like saturated fats, trans fats raise LDL (bad) cholesterol and lower HDL (good) cholesterol. But they also do other terrible things to your body: Trans fats elevate levels of triglycerides and lipoprotein, a trend that has been linked to heart disease; they make blood platelets stickier than usual and so more likely to form clots inside blood vessels in the heart, brain, and elsewhere. The latest research also shows that trans fats cause inflammation, an over activity of the immune system that plays key roles in developing heart disease, diabetes, and probably other leading causes of death and disability.

In January 2006 it became law in the U.S. that trans-fats of 0.5g or more have to be specifically listed on food labels (right beneath saturated fats). Caution: This federal law does not cover food sold in restaurants.

Chapter 7

Carbohydrates

Low Carbohydrate Diets

On a par with lumping all fats together as "bad," lumping all carbohydrates together as "bad" is an equally dangerous oversimplification. Some carbohydrates are definitely poor choices if eaten frequently because 1) they are digested quickly and rapidly release glucose (blood sugar) into the bloodstream, almost as quickly as if they were injected with a syringe, or 2) they contain few if any nutrients, adding only empty calories to pack on weight. These are carbohydrates from white bread, white rice, and pasta; highly processed foods, and sugary foods, including cake, candy, sodas, fruit juices (eating the fruit is healthier; it has fiber), and honey.

Carbohydrates are an essential part of a healthy diet. They provide the fuel we need for physical activity, mental activity, and organ function. The best sources of carbohydrates are fruits, vegetables, and whole grains. These provide essential vitamins and minerals, fiber, and important phytonutrients.

In the early 1970s, Dr. Robert Atkins introduced the popular Atkins Diet. He advocated a low-carbohydrate diet that condoned eating unrestricted amounts of protein and fat (except for trans fats), while restricting carbohydrates, particularly sugar, flour, and high-fructose corn syrups (HFCS), thus rejecting the USDA's food pyramid. His logic was that to lose weight one had to switch the body's metabolism from burning glucose to burning stored fat. The process, called *lipolysis*, begins when the body enters the state of *ketosis,* due to running out of excess carbohydrates to burn—a dangerous state for a diabetic, who shouldn't consider such a diet. It can also pose problems for those with kidney disease or with high blood pressure.

Just about every medical group and nutritional expert in America labeled the Atkins Diet an unhealthy fad—some suggesting the good doctor should be brought to task for malpractice. Now, after 25 years of Americans growing fat and unhealthy eating the unhealthy carbohydrates that the USDA food pyramid encouraged, we know Atkins had it half right, the half about eliminating the rapidly digested and non-nourishing carbohydrates. People following the diet do lose weight, but over time most gain it back as their bodies seem to sense the loss of essential micronutrients and dieters invariably go back to eating carbohydrates. What it comes down to is that it's the selection of carbohydrates that's important. And that's the rub as far as the government is concerned. Neither the United States Department of Agriculture nor the Food and Drug Administration is ever going to recommend that you boycott certain foods, whether good or bad. Agribusiness and the food factories have the political power to eat these politicians alive.

Although Dr. Atkins died in 2003, his diet is still around and popular. He was updating it when he died. It's now a more balanced diet that allows more fruits, vegetables, and whole grains but still allows almost unlimited fats.

The balanced approach of healthy carbohydrates, proteins, fats, and exercise that the Healthy Eating Pyramid recommends is now the basis of many other popular commercial diets, including the South Beach Diet, The Zone, and Nutrisystem. Americans are spending over $40 billion a year on diet programs, books, and products. It's a giant industry.

Low-Energy-Density Diets

Some diet books weight heavily on eating foods with high volumes and low calories; the logic being that foods high in water and fiber tend to fill you up and satisfy hunger. This is both true and false. Most of what you eat is water in any event, and water should be your first choice of beverage. Water is essential for digestion and kidney function. It's said that we need eight, eight ounce glasses of water a day depending on physical activity and temperature. In reality we get a great deal of that from food so we don't need to drink that much. Plus, the water in your coffee, tea, or diet soda counts as well.

It's a balancing act. Calories from fat and protein take much longer to digest into blood sugar than calories from carbohydrates; they stay in your stomach longer and also satisfy hunger. It's one of the reasons that the early Atkins Diet worked. So drinking like a camel and eating raw fiber like a termite really isn't a viable stand-alone diet plan.

Yet high volume, low calorie carbohydrates can be helpful in cutting total calorie intake. I find a cup of low calorie soup eaten before lunch makes it easier to eat smaller portions. I eat raw carrots and celery a great deal, they're mostly water with good nutrients. I've even switched from big juicy olives in my martini (on the rocks to add water) to a big stalk of cold celery on the side. The celery helps full my stomach and dilutes the booze—I get plenty of olive oil on my salads and from cooking.

Types of Carbohydrates

The abundant forms of carbohydrates are sugars, fibers, and starches.

The basic chemical component of every carbohydrate is a single sugar molecule—a simple union of carbon, hydrogen, and oxygen atoms. Starches and fibers are essentially chains of sugar molecules; some contain hundreds of sugars. Some chains are straight, others branch wildly.

Nutritionists once grouped carbohydrates into two main categories. Simple carbohydrates included sugars such as fruit sugar (fructose), corn or grape sugar (dextrose or glucose), and table sugar (sucrose). Complex carbohydrates were thought to be better for you, while sugars weren't so great. It's turned out to be more complicated than that—now they talk of glycemic index and glycemic load.

The digestive system breaks down carbohydrates (or tries to break them down) into single sugar molecules—they are the only ones small enough to cross into the bloodstream. It also converts most digestible carbohydrates into glucose (also known as blood sugar), because cells are designed to use this as a universal energy source.

Fiber is an exception—it can't be broken down into sugar molecules, and passes through the body undigested. Fiber comes as either soluble in water, or insoluble. Although fiber is not a nutrient, it is important for good health. Soluble fiber binds to fatty substances in the intestines and carries them out as waste, thus helping to lower low-density lipoproteins (LDL). Insoluble fiber helps push food through the intestinal track and helps prevent constipation.

Blood Sugar (Glucose) and Type 2 Diabetes

Your body performs best when your blood sugar is kept relatively constant. If your blood sugar drops too low, you become lethargic and/ or experience hunger. If it drops far enough you can lose consciousness and die. That's why diabetics carry sugar pills as a precaution against improper dosing of medication. Your brain uses about 20 percent of your food calories to function—no glucose no function.

The way your body controls blood glucose is really quite elegant. Glucose enters your body whenever you eat foods containing carbohydrates. Glucose levels are regulated by insulin, a hormone produced by the pancreas. When glucose levels rise, your brain signals the pancreas to secret more insulin. The insulin brings your blood sugar back down, but primarily by converting the excess sugar to stored fat. The greater the rate of increase in your blood sugar, the more chance that your body will release an excess amount of insulin, and drive your blood sugar down too low.

Sensing low blood sugar levels, the brain will then signal your pancreas to release another hormone called glucagon, which then engages the liver to release more glucose both from storage and by having it released from fat cells.

It can be a wild cycle of feeling an initial surge of energy and mood as your blood sugar rises, followed by a cycle of increased fat storage, lethargy, and more hunger. That's when you reach for a candy bar or a sugared soft drink to keep the cycle going.

The link between obesity and type 2 diabetes is indisputable. According to the Center for Disease Control (CDC) in 2005, 20.8 million people—7.3 percent of the population—had diabetes. Fewer than 10 percent of diabetics suffer from type 1 diabetes, which occurs when the body cannot produce insulin. All the rest diagnosed are type 2, the result of impaired glucose metabolism.

The American Diabetes Association considers normal blood glucose levels to be in the normal range after fasting, without exercise, to be between 70 to 110 mg/dl. [That's about one to two teaspoons for your entire blood volume of about 5 liters.] A diagnosis of diabetes is made if your blood glucose level is higher than 126 mg/dl after two consecutive blood tests.

Complications of Diabetes in the U.S. (Center for Disease Control)
Heart Disease and Stroke
+ Heart disease and stroke account for about 65% of deaths in people with diabetes.
+ Adults with diabetes have heart disease death rates about 2 to 4 times higher than adults without diabetes.
+ The risk of stroke is 2 to 4 times higher among people with diabetes.

High Blood Pressure
+ About 73% of adults with diabetes have blood pressure greater than or equal to 130/80 or use prescription medications for hypertension.

Blindness
+ Diabetes is the leading cause of new cases of blindness among adults aged 20-74.
+ Diabetic retinopathy causes 12,000 to 24,000 new cases of blindness each year.

Kidney Disease
- Diabetes is the leading cause of kidney failure, accounting for 44% of new cases in 2002.
- In 2002, 44,000 people with diabetes began treatment for end-stage kidney disease in the United States and Puerto Rico.
- In 2002, a total of 153,730 people with end-stage kidney disease due to diabetes were living on chronic dialysis or with a kidney transplant.

Nervous System Disease
- About 60% to 70% of people with diabetes have mild to severe forms of nervous damage. The results of such damage include impaired sensation or pain in the feet or hands, slowed digestion of food in the stomach, carpal tunnel syndrome, and other nerve problems.
- Almost 30% of people with diabetes aged 40 years or older have impaired sensation in the feet.
- Severe forms of diabetic nerve disease are a major contributing cause of lower-extremity amputations.

Amputations
- More than 60% of nontraumatic lower-limb amputations occur in people with diabetes.
- In 2002, about 82,000 nontraumatic lower-limb amputations were performed in people with diabetes.

Dental Disease
- Periodontal (gum) disease is more common in people with diabetes. Among young adults, those with diabetes have about twice the risk of those without diabetes.
- Almost one-third of people with diabetes have loss of attachment of the gums to the teeth measuring 5 millimeters or more.

Complications of Pregnancy
- Poorly controlled diabetes before conception and during the first trimester of pregnancy can cause birth defects in 5% to 10% of pregnancies and spontaneous abortions in 15% to 20% of pregnancies.
- Poorly controlled diabetes during the second and third trimesters of pregnancies can result in excessively large babies, posing a risk to both mother and child.

Other Complications
- Uncontrolled diabetes often leads to biochemical imbalances that can cause life-threatening events, such as diabetic ketoacidosis and hyperosmolar (nonketotic) coma.
- People with diabetes are more susceptible to many other illnesses and often have worse prognoses. For example, they are more likely to die with pneumonia or influenza than people who do not have diabetes.

Diabetes is a hidden killer. By the time you have symptoms of high blood sugar you can be in serious trouble. I have a friend who like many Americans never went to the doctor for regular checkups. One day he developed a sore on his foot, brought about by an ill-fitting boot. Trouble was it didn't heal. The outcome was a diagnosis of acute type 2 diabetes. He'd already suffered major damage to his eyes and organs, and lost that leg to gangrene. At this point he's not given very long to live—a tragedy that could have been avoided with a simple blood test.

Unfortunately, most health insurance policies, including Medicare and Medicaid, do not pay for checkups, only for treatment. It's crazy and it's bankrupting the healthcare system. Covered or not, if you care about your health you should have an annual checkup. As an airline pilot I was required to have one every six months, and checking blood sugar was always part of it.[3]

Glycemic Index – Glycemic Load

At this point we know that to lose weight or maintain a healthy weight we have to satisfy that old equation: to maintain weight energy (calories) in must = energy out; to lose weight we have to tip the equation by eating fewer calories and/or increasing physical activity. That includes all food calories, including those from fat, protein, and carbohydrates. However, when it comes to controlling the level of glucose in the blood (blood sugar) carbohydrates rule; fats and protein have little effect on blood sugar.

Carbohydrates, on the other hand, are processed into glucose at wildly different rates, which was a complete surprise to scientists when they finally got around to measuring it. White bread, for instance, floods the blood stream with glucose faster eating raw sucrose (table sugar), thus blowing away the simple/complex carbohydrate theory.

So to be healthy and avoid being overweight, and to avoid type 2 diabetes, we need to know the effect different foods containing carbohydrates have on blood sugar levels.

The earliest known work on Glycemic Index (GI) was in 1981, done by Dr. David Jenkins and associates at St. Michael's Hospital in Toronto, Canada. They tested 62 commonly eaten foods. More recent efforts to expand the Index have been made by Jennie Brand-Miller and her associates at the Human Nutrition Unit of the University of Sydney, Australia. The list is now up to about 1,600 foods—quite a task requiring at least ten volunteers to fast overnight, then eat the tested food (an amount of food that contains 50 grams of the tested carbohydrate) and have their blood sugar levels tested frequently for two hours. The scientists compare this exercise to the subject's response to a reference food, which may be liquid glucose or white bread. Since people digest at different rates multiple volunteers are used and the average indexed. Then, they repeat the whole process on different days to reduce the effect of day-to-day variations. You can access the Sydney GI database at: www.glycemicindex.com/

The theory behind the Glycemic Index is simply to minimize insulin-related problems by identifying and avoiding foods that have the greatest effect on your blood sugar.

Other factors that influence how quickly the carbohydrates in food raise blood sugar, these from HSPH, include:

- *Type of starch.* Starch comes in many different configurations. Some are easier to break into sugar molecules than others. The starch in potatoes, for example, is digested and absorbed into the bloodstream relatively quickly.

- *Fiber content.* The sugars in fiber are linked in ways that the body has trouble breaking. The more fiber a food has, the less digestible carbohydrate, and so the less sugar, it can deliver.
- *Ripeness.* Ripe fruits and vegetables tend to have more sugar than unripe ones, and so tend to have a higher glycemic index.
- *Fat and acid content.* The more fat or acid a food or meal contains, the slower its carbohydrates are converted to sugar and absorbed into the bloodstream.
- *Physical form.* Finely ground grain is more rapidly digested, and so has a higher glycemic index, than more coarsely ground grain.

Useful as Glycemic Index is it does not tell us how much digestible carbohydrate a food delivers. For example, the handful of baby carrots I enjoy has a high glycemic index but a minimal effect on my blood sugar because the carbohydrate itself is less than 1 percent of the content of the food. The rest is water. Even a small piece of candy with a high glycemic index has little effect on blood sugar levels because of the small amount eaten.

So an important extension of the Glycemic Index (GI) is the Glycemic Load (GL) that takes the quantity of the carbohydrate in the food into account. Once again, Dr. Walter Willett and his associates at the Harvard School of Public Health step to the fore. They developed this concept as early as 1997, developed it further in his fore mentioned book, and have published many of the Glycemic Load numbers.

Once you know the glycemic index (GI) you can calculate the glycemic load (GL) by multiplying the amount of carbohydrate actually consumed: GL = GI/100 x Net Carbs.

The glycemic index and glycemic load offer information about how a food affects blood sugar and insulin. The lower the GI or GL, the less the food affects blood sugar and insulin levels. A GI below 55 is considered low; a GL below 10 is considered low, below 19 high, and above 20 high.

Although it is called "blood sugar," sugars other than glucose are found in the blood, such as fructose and galactose. Only glucose levels are regulated by insulin and glucagon.

Here are Glycemic Indexes and Glycemic Loads some commonly eaten foods:

Food	GI	Serving Size	Net Carbs	GL
Peanuts	14	4 oz (113g)	15	2
Bean Spouts	25	1 cup (104g)	4	1
Grapefruit	25	½ large (166g)	11	3
Pizza	30	2 slices (260g)	42	13
Lowfat yogurt	33	1 cup (245g)	47	16
Apples	38	1 med (138)	16	6
Pasta	48	1 cup (140g)	38	16
Carrots	47	1 large (72g)	5	2
Oranges	48	1 med (131g)	12	6
Banana	52	1 large (136g)	27	14
Potato Chips	54	4 oz (114g)	55	30
Snickers Bar	55	1 bar (113g)	64	35
Brown Rice	55	1 cup (195g)	42	23
Honey	55	1 tbsp (21g)	17	9
Oatmeal	58	1 cup (234g)	21	12
Ice Cream	61	1 cup (72g)	16	10
Mac & Cheese	64	(166g)	47	30
Raisins	64	(43g)	32	20
White Rice	64	1 cup (186g)	52	33
Sucrose	68	1 tbsp	12	8
White Bread	70	1 slice (30g)	14	10
Watermelon	72	1 cup (154g)	11	8
Popcorn	72	2 cups (16g)	10	7
Baked Potato	85	1 med (173g)	33	28
Glucose	100	(50g)	50	50

Chapter 8

Protein

The last of the macronutrients joining fats and carbohydrates is protein. What is protein? Well, it's you—take away the water and you're about 75 percent protein. It's in muscle, bone, skin, hair, and every other body part or tissue. It's the enzymes that power many chemical reactions and the hemoglobin that carries oxygen in your blood. There are at least 10,000 different proteins that make and keep you what you are.

About twenty basic building blocks, called amino acids, provide the raw material for all proteins. Following instructions from your genes, the body strings together amino acids; some short, some long, some that fold, and others that are three-dimensional structures. [Genes contain the instructions for the production of proteins, which make up the structure of cell. Each human has an estimated 90,000 genes.]

Your body is constantly rebuilding itself. Because the body doesn't store amino acids, it needs a fresh supply of protein every day—in essence you need protein from food to make your own body's protein. The good news is the body doesn't need much protein from food to do it. We need about 7 grams of protein for every 20 pounds of lean body weight; for a 150-pound person that's slightly over 70 grams daily for an adult. Beyond that, the science as to what kinds of proteins is at best, pretty weak according to Dr. Willett.

In the United States and other developed countries getting your minimum daily requirement of protein is easy. You can get 70 grams of protein by having cereal with milk for breakfast, a peanut butter and jelly sandwich for lunch, and a piece of fish with a side of beans for dinner. It doesn't take much. In other places in the world millions of people can't get enough protein. Protein malnutrition leads to the condition known as Kwashiorkor, which can lead to growth failure, loss of muscle mass, decreased immunity, weakening of the heart and respiratory system, and death.

As mentioned earlier, you can get too much protein from following a low-carbohydrate or no-carbohydrate diet. Robbed of carbohydrates to burn, the body enters the state of *ketosis,* which is very dangerous for those with diabetes, kidney disease, or high blood pressure. Also, digesting protein releases acids that the body neutralizes with calcium. Eating a lot of protein over time takes a lot of calcium that may be pulled from bone. Tracking a very large group, the Nurses Health Study showed that those eating 95 grams of protein a day over a 12-year period were 20 percent more likely to have broken a wrist then those who ate 68 grams or less.

Vegetarians and Vegans

Some of the proteins you eat contain all of the amino acids needed to build new protein; these are called complete proteins—animal sources of protein tend to be complete. Incomplete proteins from fruits, vegetables, grains, and nuts may lack one or more amino acids that the body can't make or create by modifying another amino acid.

Vegetarians and vegans need to be extremely cautious. Those who don't eat meat, fish, poultry, eggs, or dairy products need to eat a variety of other protein-containing foods each day.

Animal protein and vegetable protein seem to have the same effects on health. But how the protein is packaged makes a huge difference— food doesn't ever come as protein alone, unless from chemistry. For instance, a juicy 6-ounce porterhouse steak has tons of protein, 38 grams, but it also provides 44 grams of fat, 16 of them saturated. The same amount of halibut has 44 grams of protein with less than 1 gram of saturated fat, and more than 4 grams of polyunsaturated and monounsaturated fats that you need.

Long maligned, eggs aren't a bad choice either. Although the egg yolks have a lot of cholesterol, the entire egg is low in saturated fat, plenty of protein (over 6 grams an egg), vitamins B12 and D, riboflavin, and folic acid and only 90 calories. Now most nutritionists suggest that people who don't have a high cholesterol problem eat up to three eggs a week. My wife and I enjoy a few eggs at Sunday brunch—usually with some wine or a Bloody Mary.

So it's important to pay attention to what your protein comes with. If you're at McDonald's or other fast food restaurants forget it; you're going to get saturated fats, and loads of calories along with your protein. Your best choices are lean cuts of beef, skinned poultry, fish, and vegetable proteins, beans, nuts, and whole grains. I personally find staying away from cheese important—it's high in saturated fat and calories. Now I have some low-fat yogurt or low-fat cottage cheese. As for milk, the USDA's recommendation of three glasses a day is ludicrous, unless you're a calf. If you use milk on cereal, use skim milk, you'll get the protein with less fat.

Follows is a list of foods with protein provided by the USDA:

Food	Serving	Protein grams
Hamburger, lean	6 oz (170g)	48.6
Chicken, roasted	6 oz (170g)	42.5
Fish	6 oz (170g)	41.2
Tuna, in water	6 oz (170g)	40.1
Beefsteak, broiled	6 oz (170g)	38.6
Cottage cheese	1 cup (225g)	28.1
Cheese pizza	2 slices (128g)	15.4
Yogurt, low fat	8 oz (227g)	11.9
Tofu	½ cup (126g)	10.1
Lentils, cooked	½ cup (99g)	9
Skim milk	1 cup (245g)	8.4

Split peas	½ cup (98g)	8.1
Whole milk	1 cup (244g)	8
Lentil soap	1 cup (242g)	7.8
Kidney beans	½ cup (87g)	7.6
Cheddar cheese	1 oz (28g)	7.1
Macaroni	1 cup (140g)	6.8
Soymilk	1 cup (245g)	6.7
Egg	1 lg (50g)	6.3
Whole wheat bread	2 slices (56g)	5.4
White bread	2 slices (60g)	4.9
Rice	1 cup (158g)	4.3
Broccoli	5 inch piece (140g)	4.2
Baked potato	2"x5" (156g)	3
Corn	1 ear (77g)	2.6

Chapter 9

The Micronutrients

Micronutrients are the essential organic components of foods, such as vitamins, which are present in very small amounts that enable the body to function normally. Unlike macronutrients (fats, carbohydrates, and protein) that your body breaks down by digestion, micronutrients are absorbed without being broken down—that's why your body only needs small amounts and why large amounts can be toxic.

Lurking in the background to pick your pocket is the giant dietary supplement industry. In 2007, wholesale, retail, and mail-order sales were reported by Nutraceuticals World to be $30 billion in the United States; globally sales are expected to reach $187 billion by 2010. The products sold include, vitamins, herbal and botanicals, sports nutrition products, meal supplements, minerals, and specialty supplements. The top health categories for supplements are weight loss, heart problems, digestion, arthritis or joint pain, seasonal allergies, vision and eye health, and diabetes—mostly sales to people suffering from chronic disease who are reaching out for an easy cure.

The use of foods for medicinal value goes back far longer than modern medicine. Some that have been accepted as healing are pretty bizarre. In Chinese traditional medicine, animal parts—known in East Asia as *pu foods*—are reputed to endow a man with the potency of the animal itself, or with the potency implied by the shape of the appendage. Rhinoceros horns and tiger penises are particularly sought for that purpose making these animals' critically endangered species. Due to poaching, Caspian, Bali, and Java tigers are already considered extinct. Can Viagra and other erectile dysfunction (ED) drugs make a difference in the market for animal parts? Perhaps, but ED drugs are expensive costing $8 to $10 a pill, but, then again a bowl of tiger penis soup sells for $350 in the black markets of Hong Kong, South Korea, and Taiwan. Go figure.

How well does the United States Food and Drug Administration (FDA) regulate the dietary supplement industry? Most experts don't think the FDA regulates it well enough to prevent people from dangerously self-medicating. The information regarding vitamin supplements is particularly confusing and frustrating. Not many years ago most experts would tell you that taking vitamins just made expensive urine and was a waste of money. Today they're not so sure that some vitamins taken above the minimum daily requirement might not help prevent heart disease, cancer, osteoporosis, and other chronic diseases. Others think that additional vitamins, particularly vitamin E and bet-carotene could make those diseases worse.

Certainly, getting the minimum daily requirement of vitamins is prudent for most people; folic acid, and vitamins B_6, B_{12}, D, and E can be difficult to get only from food unless your daily diet is selected with great care. Strict vegetarians and vegans need to be particularly careful because vitamin B_{12} is found only in animal products. Eating plenty of fruits, vegetables, and whole grains is still your best bet, but a one-a-day vitamin supplement may be a good insurance policy. If you have precancerous growths or cancer you should check with your doctor before taking any vitamin supplement, or you could wind up feeding a cancer. According to the latest medical advice, mega-dosing on antioxidants like vitamins A, C, and E may also be harmful.

We need more hard science concerning micronutrients. The nutrition (fertilizers and animal feed) put into the food chain by the factory farms is focused on the quantity of the food produced, not the quality of the nutrients passed on to us. Our health depends on those nutrients, so as the pressure on world food supplies increases it's going to be important that the quality of those nutrients is not compromised. Basically, if the plants don't get fed right we don't either. (see afterward for more)

Vitamins are usually classified as fat-soluble or water-soluble. Fat-soluble vitamins (A, D, E, and K) are stored in the liver and fatty tissues and transported by blood lipids—it's one of the reasons we need plenty of the good fats in our diet. Because fat-soluble vitamins are stored for long periods taking megadoses of them can be toxic and lead to health problems.

Water-soluble vitamins (C and the B-complex) are not stored; these are eliminated by the body quickly. These need regular replacement, preferably through nutritious food.

Antioxidants

Prior to the 1990s only chemists and nutritional researchers had even heard the word. That changed when the diet supplement industry stated promoting vitamins A, C, E, and beta carotene as antioxidants and Americans responded by gobbling up vast quantities.

While scientists agree that "free radicals" (oxygen based by-products of oxygen-using reactions like those to burn fat and carbohydrates) are connected to heart disease, cancer, diabetes, Alzheimer's and Parkinson's disease, there is no real evidence that shows that taking antioxidant supplements is an effective therapy. Recent scientific studies have shown, however, that mega doses of antioxidants can be extremely harmful. If you're a smoker, beta carotene can increase the risk of developing lung cancer. Even scarier is scientific speculation that mega doses of vitamin E may even increase the risk of early death.

Clearly, the safest bet is to eat a heart-healthy diet, which will contain plenty of natural antioxidants, exercise, and even enjoy a moderate amount of alcohol. It's better for you than popping pills.

Vitamin A

Vitamin A is also known as retinol, retinaldehyde, and retinoic acid. Just like mother told you, eating carrots will help you see in the dark. Well, not really, but carrots do contain a lot of beta carotene, which is broken down in the small intestine to retinol, a form of vitamin A. And it is good for your eyes and the health of those cells lining the body's interior surfaces. It also stimulates the production of white blood cells and takes part in remodeling bones. Many fruits and vegetables contain beta-carotene, and other vitamin A precursors that the body can turn into vitamin A. Also, many breakfast cereals, juices and dairy products, are fortified with vitamin A—so you're probably getting plenty of it. Vitamin A is fat-soluble. The recommended daily intake of vitamin A is 700 micrograms for women and 900 micrograms for men. Caution, the upper limit is 3,000 micrograms.

Vitamin B

There are eight B vitamins. Two we've already talked about; vitamin B_1, thiamin, prevents us from getting beriberi; and vitamin B_3 niacin, prevents us from getting pellagra. All of the B vitamins are water-soluble. The recommended daily intake of vitamin B_1 is 1.1 milligrams for women and 1.2 milligrams for men; vitamin B_3 is 1.1 milligrams for women and 1.3 milligrams for men. The upper limits for both vitamins are not known.

Note: Some vitamins are dosed in micrograms, others in milligrams. 1 milligram (mg) is equal to 1,000 micrograms (mcg).

Vitamin B9, or folic acid

Over thirty years ago, British researchers found that mothers of children with spina bifida had low vitamin levels. Spina bifida is a birth defect that involves the incomplete development of the spinal cord or its coverings. With that knowledge, two large trials were conducted in which women were randomly assigned to take folic acid (the form of folate added to multivitamins or fortified foods) or a placebo—the study showed that getting too little folate increased a women's chance of having a baby with spina bifida or anencephaly and that getting enough folate could prevent these defects. Anencephaly is a defect in the closure of the neural tube to the brain during fetal development. Both of these defects, spina bifida and anencephaly, usually occurs during the third and fourth week of pregnancy. To be effective, folate must be taken either before conception or in the few weeks after.

The problem is that getting enough folate, at least 400 micrograms, from food alone can be difficult. In 1992, the Centers for Disease Control and Prevention (CDC) recommended that all women who could become pregnant take 400 micrograms of folic acid a day. Recognizing that women were not heeding their advice, the Food and Drug Administration now requires that folic acid be added to most enriched breads, flour, cornmeal, pastas, rice, and other grain products, along with the iron, and other micronutrients that have been added for years.

Current research into the role vitamin, B_9 (folic acid), B_6, and B_{12} in helping to prevent heart disease and cancer are actively under way. There are many indications that they do this by helping to recycle artery-clogging homocysteine (an amino acid) into other harmless amino acids. According to the American Heart Association, "Epidemiological studies have shown that too much homocysteine in the blood (plasma) is related to a higher risk of coronary heart disease, stroke and peripheral vascular disease. Other evidence suggests that homocysteine may have an effect on atherosclerosis by damaging the inner lining of arteries and promoting blood clots. However, a direct causal link hasn't been established."

The disappointing data are that only a fraction of U.S. adults get the recommended daily intake of all the B vitamins by diet alone. The data reinforces the fact that one can be overweight and undernourished—65 percent of U.S. adults are overweight. So use of a daily multivitamin is an important safeguard for most of us. The B-complex vitamins are water-soluble.

The recommended daily intake:

Vitamin B_9 (folic acid) is 400 micrograms. The upper limit is 1,000 micrograms.

Vitamin B_6 (pyridoxal, pyridoxine, pyridoxamine) is between 1.3 and 1.7 milligrams; larger men and those over 51 should have slightly more. The upper limit is 100 milligrams.

Vitamin B_{12} (cobalamin) is 2.4 micrograms. The upper limit is not known.

Vitamin C

Although vitamin C wasn't discovered until 1932, for centuries before it was known that citrus fruits could cure or prevent scurvy, a disease that routinely killed early sailors on long journeys away from fresh foods.

In the 1970s, Chemistry and Peace Nobel laureate Linus Pauling received national and worldwide attention by strongly promoting mega doses of vitamin C (citrus acid). He claimed that taking an amount of vitamin C equivalent to 12 to 24 oranges was a way to ward off colds and potentially other chronic diseases. While there's no question that vitamin C plays a role in fighting infections, and is needed to make collagen, a tissue needed to make bones, teeth, gums, and blood vessels, there's absolutely no clinical evidence that getting mega doses of vitamin C will prevent colds or other diseases. On the other hand, a vitamin C deficiency can make you vulnerable to infectious diseases.

Vitamin C is water-soluble. The recommended daily intake of vitamin C is 90 milligrams for men and 75 milligrams for women—add 35 milligrams for smokers.

Vitamin D

Sunshine: you need it just like your plants. Sounds easy, but it's not. It's estimated that 1 billion people worldwide have inadequate levels of vitamin D in their blood. I remember as a young pilot on a transoceanic stop in Iceland during the time that the sun once again began rising in the northern Polar Regions, being amazed at people sunbathing, in fairly cold temperatures; they simple knew their bodies needed vitamin D, which had been lacking during the time of perpetual darkness.

When one thinks of osteoporosis we immediately focus on calcium, yet calcium without vitamin D has proved to be valueless. We need both. Without vitamin D the body cannot absorb and retain calcium and phosphorus that are both necessary to build bone. Also, scientific studies have shown that vitamin D keeps cancer cells from growing, and plays an essential role in controlling infections. Extreme and prolonged vitamin D deficiency can cause rickets, the softening and weakening of bones in children.

Statistically, a great many Americans are vitamin D deficient. You may be too.

Very few foods contain vitamin D. Good sources are dairy products and breakfast cereals, both of which are fortified with vitamin D, and fatty fish, which I happen to love.

Vitamin D is fat-soluble. The Institute of Medicine's current recommended intake of vitamin D is 5 micrograms (200 IU) up to age 50, 10 micrograms (400 IU) between ages 51 and 70, and 51 micrograms (600 IU) after that. Optimal intakes are much higher, with at least 25 to 50 micrograms (1,000 to 2,000 IU) recommended for those over age 2.

Caution, while extremely high doses vitamin D (hundreds of thousands of IU) can be toxic and even deadly, taking up to 2,000 IU is considered safe for an adult.

Vitamin E

Early studies, including the Nurses' Health Study and the Health Professional Follow-up Study, seem to indicate a 20 percent to 40 percent reduction in coronary heart disease for men and women who took at least 100 IU for at least two years. [100 IU of synthetic vitamin E is about 90 milligrams (mg)] Subsequent studies, including the Heart Outcomes Prevention Evaluation (HOPE), however, showed no benefit of four years worth of vitamin E supplementation among 9,500 men and women who had been diagnosed with heart disease or at high risk for it. Based on the HOPE study and others, the American Heart Association has concluded, "The scientific data do not justify the use of antioxidant vitamin supplements [such as vitamin E] for CVD risk reduction."

In 2005, an analysis of the vitamin E trial was released. It concluded that users of high-dose vitamin E (more than 400 IU per day) might have a slightly higher death rate than non-users. Although that press release got quite a lot of notoriety, the Institute of Medicine found vitamin E was safe at much higher doses. So who knows? Maybe we'll get better guidance in the future.

My wife and I play it safe by taking a one-a-day vitamin and mineral supplement that contains vitamin E at 50 IU, and by eating lots of vegetable oil on our dark green leafy salads, and eating fish. I particularly like good oily herring.

Vitamin E is fat-soluble. The Institute of Medicine recommends a daily intake of 15 mg of vitamin E from food, the equivalent of 33 IU in synthetic form. The upper limit, they conclude, getting more than 1,000 milligrams of supplemental vitamin E is not safe; that's about 2,200 IU of synthetic vitamin E.

Vitamin K

Vitamin K is a fat-soluble vitamin that helps make six of the thirteen proteins needed for blood clotting. If you've ever had to take anticoagulants such as warfarin (Coumadin) you know all about vitamin K because of your doctor's warning not to over eat green leafy vegetables, or take a daily vitamin supplement. I know about warfarin and vitamin K because of a phlebitis episode that sent clots up to my lungs. If you're on an anticoagulant, too much vitamin K will reverse the effect of warfarin to increase clotting. I was grounded for six months because the FAA won't allow an airline pilot to fly while on Coumadin therapy.

Recently, researchers have discovered that vitamin K joins vitamin D in being involved with building bone. Low levels of vitamin K in the bloodstream have been linked with low bone density, and when given supplements of vitamin K bone strength improved. Information gathered by the Nurses Health Study suggests that women who don't get much vitamin K are twice as likely to break a hip, compared to women who get plenty.

The current recommendation for vitamin K is that men should have a daily intake of 120 micrograms and women 90 micrograms. If you don't eat green leafy vegetables regularly and commonly used cooking oils, chances are you're vitamin K deficient. National data indicates that only 1 in 4 Americans meet the goal for vitamin K from food alone.

Calcium and Milk

While just about everyone knows that calcium is important for strong bones, if you heeded the dairy industries advertisements you'd be drinking milk like a calf. But guess what, there are plenty of ways to get enough calcium in your diet and avoid some of the unhealthy sides of overloading with milk and other dairy products. The USDA's Dietary Guidelines, 2005, goes as far as recommending three glasses of milk a Day! In *Eat, Drink, and Be Healthy,* Dr. Willett writes that there are six reasons why you shouldn't be conned into using large amounts of it: lactose intolerance, saturated fat, extra calories, unneeded hormones, a possible risk of prostate cancer, and a possible increased risk of ovarian cancer."

- *Lactose intolerance.* Although all babies are born able to digest milk that ability is lost as we grow older and stop making an enzyme called lactase that breaks down milk sugar. Lactose intolerance is far from rare; only a quarter of the world's population can fully digest milk. In the United States, about fifty million of us can't digest milk. My wife Sue is lactose intolerant. If she drinks milk or eats more than a small amount of ice cream, she gets nauseous, bloated, cramps, and diarrhea. Lactose-modified milk is available, and powders and tablets to be taken before eating dairy products can help you digest it—but the fact remains you don't need to force yourself to do so just to get calcium.

- *Saturated fat.* A glass of whole milk has almost 5 grams of saturated fat, about 20 percent of the 20-gram recommended limit. If you drink three glasses, as the USDA recommends, you'll have gotten almost your whole daily allotment—the equivalent of twelve pieces of bacon or a Big Mac and an order of French fries. True, drinking skimmed milk is much better, providing you don't eat the fat that's been skimmed off in other foods like premium ice creams and high fat snack foods.

- *Extra calories.* Three glasses of whole milk a day is 450 calories or a quarter of the average person's daily allotment. Even low-fat milk is 330 calories. It's way too much if your only goal is get more calcium.

- *Extra hormones.* Elsie the cow makes most of the same hormones that humans make. Farmers keep milk cows pregnant because pregnant cows produce more milk; they also produce more hormones in their milk, such as estrogens and progestins, androgens, and insulin like factors, to name a few. Estrogens and progestins can stimulate breast cancer, androgens promote prostate cancer, and elevated levels of insulin-like growth factors have been linked with breast, prostate, and colon cancer.

♦ *Prostate cancer.* Nine separate studies have shown that the most consistent dietary factor linked with prostate cancer was high consumption of milk or dairy products. In the Health Professionals Follow-up Study, men who drank two or more glasses of milk a day were almost twice as likely to develop advanced or metastatic prostate cancer as those who didn't drink milk at all.

Initially, researchers thought that the connection between dairy products and prostate cancer was due to the saturated fat in dairy products. But a more careful analysis of the data suggests calcium might be the reason. Men who took in more than 2,000 mg of calcium from food and supplements were almost three times as likely to develop prostate cancer and more than four times as likely to develop advanced prostate cancer as men who got less than 500 mg/day. It's thought that a high level of calcium in the body slows or even stops the conversion of inactive vitamin D into a biologically active form and thus robs the body of a natural anticancer mechanism.

The advice is that men should keep their daily intake of calcium below 1,000 mg.

♦ *Breast cancer.* Breast cancer that appears before menopause seems to be associated with high intake of full-fat dairy products. This is especially the case for estrogen-receptor positive (ER+) breast cancer, in which estrogen stimulates cancer cells to grow and divide.

♦ *Ovarian cancer.* About fifteen years ago, Harvard Medical School researchers suggested that high levels of galactose, a simple sugar released by the digestion of lactose in milk, could damage the ovary and possibly lead to ovarian cancer. Since, a number of studies have tested the hypothesis. Although the evidence isn't conclusive, a positive link between galactose and ovarian cancer shows up too many times to ignore the possibility that it may be harmful.

I learned the dark side of dairy products from researching Dr. Willett's work and Harvard School of Public Health publications; I certainly didn't know anything about it when I started my weight loss program over two years ago. When it came to milk and dairy products, my wife Sue was always cautious because of her intolerance. I, on the other hand, loved cheese and ate it very liberally and only cut back because of trying to cut calories. Now my intake of dairy products is low. I use very little milk, only some skim on cereal, eat a cup of low-fat yogurt or low-fat cottage cheese fairly frequently, enjoy a weekly bowl of onion soap (with mozzarella cheese), and a few other dairy products such as some butter and grated cheese. All of which is probably bad news for my dairy farm neighbor, and the dairy farmers across the river in Vermont. But which is more important, your health or the dairy products industry? Better to eat defensively and be healthy.

That said about dairy products and calcium, bone health and the threat of osteoporosis is an important consideration, particularly for senior citizens. Here are a few facts from the American Academy of Orthopedic Surgeons:

+ Osteoporosis is a disease of progressive bone loss associated with an increased risk of fractures. The term osteoporosis literally means porous bone. The disease often develops unnoticed over many years, with no symptoms or discomfort until a fracture occurs. Osteoporosis often causes a loss of height and dowager's hump (a severely rounded upper back).

+ Osteoporosis is a major health problem, affecting 28 million Americans and contributing to an estimated 1.5 million bone fractures per year.

+ One in two women and one in five men older than 65 years will sustain bone fractures caused by osteoporosis. Many of these painful fractures of the hip, spine, wrist, arm, and leg often occur as a result of a fall. However, performing even simple household tasks can result in a fracture of the spine it the bones have been weakened by osteoporosis.

+ The most serious and debilitating osteoporotic fracture is a hip fracture. Most patients who experience a hip fracture and previously lived independently will require help from their family or home care. All patients who experience a hip fracture will require walking aids for several months, and nearly half will permanently need canes or walkers to move around their house or outdoors. Health care costs from hip fractures total more than $10 billion annually - $35,000 per patient.[4]

The health of your bones is very serious stuff if you hope to live an independent old age. Everyone loses bone with age. After 35 years of age, the body builds less new bone to replace the loss of old bone; consequently, in general, the older you are, the lower your total bone mass and the greater your risk for osteoporosis. It's essential that senior citizens, particularly postmenopausal women, determine if they have significant bone mass loss. Your doctor can perform a safe, painless test to determine if you have a low bone density problem. If you do, there are treatments; if you don't, it's important that you develop a strategy with your doctor to avoid it.

Things beside calcium intake that influence bone growth are exercise, the sex hormones estrogen and testosterone, vitamin D, vitamin K, and fluoride. Eating a lot of animal protein can also make a difference because, as they are digested, acids are released into the blood that calcium, drawn mostly from the skeleton, helps neutralize.

Hormone replacement for women is statistically a double-edged sword. The Women's Health Initiatives study showed a large increase in breast cancer and a small but significant increase of heart disease and stroke among women who used estrogen with a progestin—there are other drug alternatives, however.

For men over age sixty-five, a testosterone check is a good idea. I was diagnosed with a very low testosterone level and prescribed a topical gel that I use daily. The only negative side effect I have is the cost of about $10 a day, which Medicare D only partly covers.

Be physically active. When it comes to bones and muscle, if you don't use it, you lose it. Just about every reliable source recommends at least a half hour of exercise a day. (See Chapter 15, Physical Activity and Exercise)

Experts advise us to take extra vitamin D (1,000-2,000 IU), and get enough vitamin K by eating at least one serving of green leafy vegetables a day. They also warn us not to get much extra preformed vitamin A (retinol) unless prescribed by a doctor, and to keep our daily dose from supplements less than 3,000 IU.

Other Mineral and Phytonutrients

In Chapter 5, I listed all of the chemical elements and minerals that the human body is composed of. Since the body is constantly rebuilding itself, we need an ongoing supply of these building blocks. We also have to respect the limits of science—there are undoubtedly other phytonutrients or bioactive components from plants that have health benefits that we don't know about. It's for that reason we need a variety of wholesome foods.

To study all the minerals we need in our diet regularly is too lengthy for here. But know that deficiencies of these essential minerals are all related to disease or health problems. Instead here are listed the ingredients of the one-a-day multivitamin/multimineral supplement my wife and I take. It's a very popular brand said to be for adults 50+, with cautions: not for children, to consult with your doctor if you are pregnant, nursing, or taking medication. And another important warning: long-term intake of high levels of vitamin A (including that sourced from beta carotene) may increase the risk of osteoporosis in adults. Do not take this product if you are using other vitamin A supplements. Mind you all the cautions are written in very small print. Anyway here they are along with the percentage of daily value (% DV):

Vitamin A	2,500 IU	50%	(40% as beta carotene)
Vitamin C	90 mg	150%	
Vitamin D	500 IU	125%	
Vitamin E	50 IU	167%	
Vitamin K	30 mcg	38%	
Thiamin	1.5 mg	100%	
Riboflavin	1.7 mg	100%	
Niacin	20 mg	100%	
Vitamin B_6	3 mg	150%	

Folic Acid	500 mcg	125%	
Vitamin B$_{12}$	25 mcg	417%	
Biotin	30 mcg	10%	
Pantothhenic Acid	10 mg	100%	
Calcium	220 mg	22%	
Phosphorus	110 mg	11%	
Iodine	150 mcg	100%	
Magnesium	50 mg	13%	
Zinc	11 mg	73%	
Selenium	55 mcg	79%	
Copper	0.9	45%	
Manganese	2.3 mg	115%	
Chromium	45 mcg	38%	
Molybdenum	45 mcg	60%	
Chloride	72 mg	2%	
Potassium	80 mg	2%	
Boron	150 mcg	*	(*DV not established)
Nickel	5 mcg	*	
Silicon	2 mg	*	
Vanadium	10 mcg	*	
Lutein	250 mcg	*	
Lycopene	300 mcg	*	

Although it seems like a huge chemical brew, it works for me. I've taken a one-a-day vitamin/mineral supplement most of my adult life. The product we're taking now is targeted for people over 50 years old. Following Dr. Willett's advice, I've recently added a separate one a day calcium (600 mg) and vitamin D (400 IU) supplement.

To determine which supplements may be right for you or other members of your family, I strongly recommend that you discuss it with your doctor. These are powerful drugs and should be treated as such.

Chapter 10

Dueling Diets

Recently, discussing my 100-pound weight loss with a large lady who hadn't seen me in awhile, she said, "that's no big deal, I've lost hundreds of pounds during my life; it just never stayed off!" Unfortunately, I think her experience is the norm for people who "diet." Getting back to the simple rule of food energy balance, any time you take in fewer calories than you burn in a day you'll have burned them from fat cells and you'll lose weight. Some people do it often with trendy, short-term diets—the trick is to keep the weight off.

Energy in/energy burned creates an extraordinary delicate balance that you can chart by weighing yourself, without clothing, at the same time of day, with an accurate scale. I've kept a record since I started my weight loss program that I update frequently. I know I'm a data freak, but if you're serious about losing weight and not regaining it you have to track your weight very closely. The minute you see the scale heading north, reduce your food intake the next day or two and increase the intensity of your activities to adjust back. That's the reason I recommend daily weight checks so it won't get ahead of you. Others say check your weight once a week. I disagree. I think a careless week could be a major setback, causing you to get discouraged and give up. Maintaining a healthy weight or losing weight requires a great deal of diligence; doing so has to be a top priority every day. It's worth the effort if you want to feel better and live a healthier, longer life.

While you can lose weight by cutting down on calories and/or by exercising more to burn those calories off, diets that leave you feeling deprived or extremely hungry don't work; eventually you'll stop doing it and gain the weight back. The reason I've named the book the *Two Martini Diet* isn't to encourage people to drink, although experts think a few drinks a day may be good for you; it's to spread the word that you can lose weight and feel good. With my weight loss strategy I have never felt I was making a great sacrifice nor have I experienced anything more than a healthy appetite, and, yes, I still enjoy my martinis.

My parents, who passed away some years ago, were working class Italian immigrants. Father and mother were always slender—heck, my father held down two or three physically demanding jobs all his working life. True, after he retired and they grew older they put on a few pounds. My grandmother died young, leaving mother to care for my grandfather and her younger brother, my uncle. She learned to cook both from her mother and from my father's mother after they married. Traditionally, that's the way people learned about what to eat and how to cook, it was passed from one generation to the next. Believe me, I never went hungry. Mother wouldn't have her only child a skinny kid. I remember when I was four or five she was particularly concerned I'd die from malnutrition and started supplementing my meals with a mixture of ginger ale and heavy cream. Don't try it, it's deadly, but delicious.

Essentially, I was raised on a modified Italian/Mediterranean diet. It was modified by the fact that we lived in Brooklyn, New York, and not in southern Italy with its warmer climate and its abundance of fresh fruits, vegetables, fish, grapes, and olives. We did have local markets that sold fresh produce from local farms in New Jersey and upstate New York, including live chickens, and both an A&P and Safeway supermarket, which were hardly super by today's standard. Mother's preference was to buy fresh vegetables from a vender with a horse-drawn cart who cruised the neighborhood once or twice a week. In contrast, most of today's produce comes from giant monoculture farms, much of it from very far away or abroad.

Born in 1937, my young diet was also affected, probably for the better, by WW II food rationing of foods like meat and butter. Mother set a great table but it tended to be high on white wheat semolina pasta and Italian bread, and white potatoes, inexpensive, high glycemic, filling foods. But she also cooked a lot of vegetables. I'll give you some of her recipes later in the next chapter. We cook them frequently. It's the dilemma of many mothers today, trying to fill bellies on limited budgets. Unfortunately, many today don't have the traditional training that my mother had and don't know the importance of vegetables and good oils.

My first wife Carol brought to our young family's table a Jewish/German tradition. We were married twenty-five years. My present wife Sue cooks foods from her childhood learned from her mother when they lived on a Baltimore-area farm where she served up Pennsylvania Dutch traditional foods. All three traditions have wonderful foods but they can be loaded with saturated fat and high glycemic load carbohydrates such as, potatoes, pasta and noodles, pies and breads—foods meant for dawn to dusk hardworking farmers, not airline pilots who sat on their duff like I did.

Fast foods and giant portions didn't help either. While my family was never junk food eaters, I always earned a good income and we had the money to eat high on the hog. We loved Chinese take-out and thought it was good for us because it has lots of vegetables. Actually, it also has food additives such as mono-sodium glutamate (MSG) that many people are allergic to and lots of white rice and noodles with a high glycemic load. Pizza was also a favorite—all that gooey mozzarella cheese had to be good for you. It was protein after all! Or so we reasoned. Some other favorite meals were giant steaks (a pound or more) with a large baked potato (with butter and/or sour cream) and a small salad on the side, or two double-thick pork chops, or several lamb chops, or Italian sausages with fried potatoes. Add in lots of processed cold cuts and white bread for lunch and you get the picture. We were eating what has become known as the deadly "Western Diet."

The Western Diet is what we've been cautioning you about throughout this book. It's a diet born of affluence, food availability at relatively low cost, and ignorance. Agribusiness, the food factories, and your government have promulgated the Western Diet and Americans have bought it hook, line, and sinker. They push red and processed meats, value added processed foods, refined grains, sweets and desserts, and high saturated fat dairy products. It's what people have been programmed to want and where the profits are.

You could work with the traditional diets from your parents and grandparents and adjust according to your caloric needs; the basics of lots of vegetables, good oils, and fruit are already part of the diet. If you grew up on the Western Diet, you don't have that in your memory bank. You have to learn to use vegetables, good oils, and fruit. You have to program yourself to simply eliminate some foods such as white bread, white potatoes, white rice, and sugared sodas, and to use others such as red and processed meats, sweets and desserts, and dairy products sparingly, and most important, to substitute whole grains for the white highly processed grains. This substitution can be made in almost all the traditional diets, and as we've learned is essential for good health.

Add to my at-home meals those that I ate on the road flying, about 50 percent of my food intake, and it's not hard to understand why my weight unrelentingly climbed throughout my career. Now almost fifty years later, at age 70, I'm about back where I started. My first airline uniform jacket was 42" around the shoulders, and I had a 36" waist; I weighed about 165 pounds. I now wear the same size jacket and have a 36$\frac{1}{2}$" waist, and weigh 167 pounds. I'm actually more muscular now than I was when I was 21-years-old with a body analyzer BMI of between 10 and 12. Take a look at my pictures.

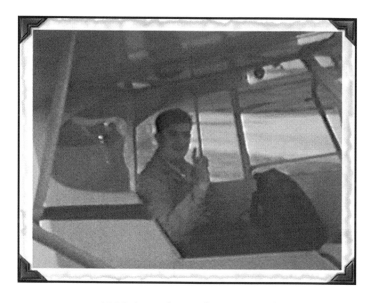

1953 A student pilot – age 16

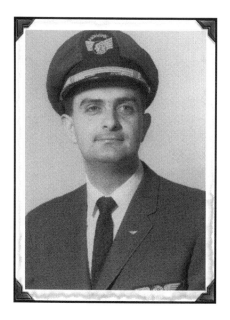

1960 A freshly minted Captain – age 23

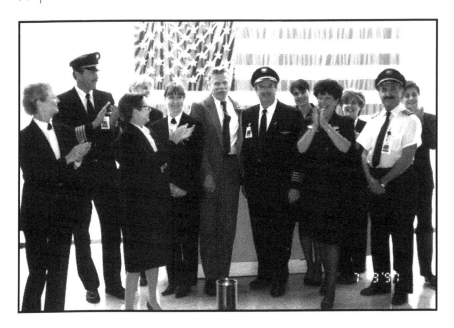

1997 Retirement celebration – age 60

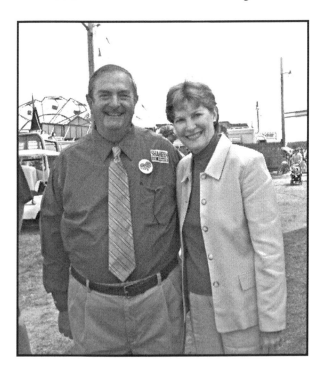

2002 On the campaign trial with Gov. Shaheen – age 65

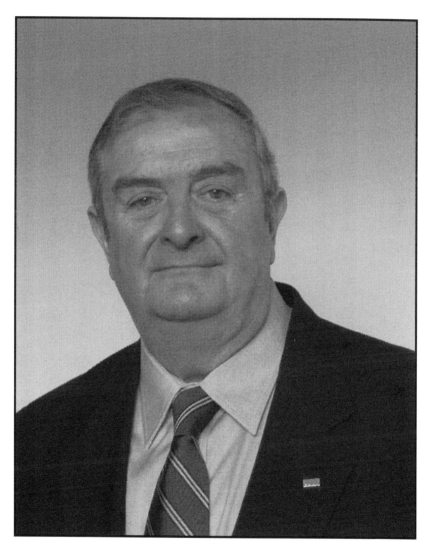

2004 Poster [2004 Senate campaign – age 67

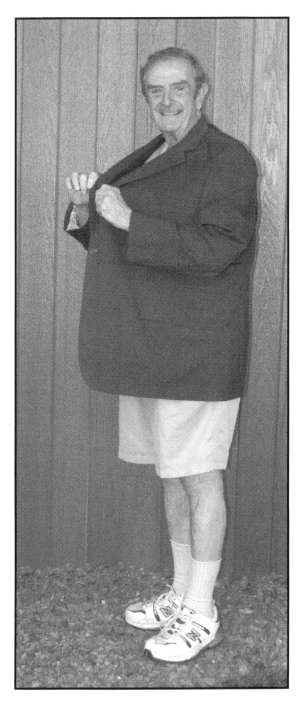

2008 clothes don't fit anymore – age 71

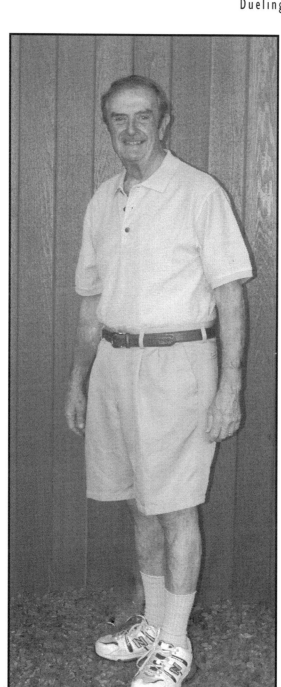

2008 102 pounds lighter

There were a few things that kept my weight from simply skyrocketing. While I enjoyed a piece of chocolate on occasion, I never was a sugar junky, never drank sugared sodas or even put sugar in my coffee, which I also drink black. That and I have always exercised. In my childhood days we played outside. There were no TVs or computers. Our favorite neighborhood game was stickball, played with a light, high bouncing, Spaulding ball and a broomstick bat. I was a great pitcher; something I feel to this day because my right shoulder hurts when the barometer is low. I was blessed with a loving family and a wonderful childhood; if you want to read more about my career as an airline pilot and my rich family life get my memoir, *A Good Stick; An Airline Captain Lives the History of 20th Century Commercial Aviation,* it's available through any book store, or accessed through my website www.Sorlucco.com

As a young man and into middle age, I used to play a lot of tennis, ski, jog, do strength-building exercises, and ride a bike. I not only enjoyed physical activity but I had a need to stay in shape because I had to pass flight physicals every six months. Back in the days when airline pilots actually had layovers with time for rest and recreation, other crewmembers and I would often bid overnights together where tennis courts were available, bring rackets and play. Now I use my home gym just about every day and do ground work outdoors. Whatever it is you enjoy doing, you have to be physically active or the fat will creep up on you and you'll grow less and less able to do anything. It's a totally unnecessary self-defeating cycle for many people, as they grow older.

When I cracked 200 pounds in my early 40s jogging became harder; by the time I turned 50 I wasn't jogging or playing tennis anymore. A fast walk was about the best I could manage. At age 66, I had to stop skiing; weighing over 250 pounds my knees and hips just couldn't take the pounding anymore. Finally, at 68, after knee surgery, at 270 pounds I made the decision of a lifetime, to lose weight and live. If you're a young person and slender don't make the mistake I made by allowing yourself to gain weight. If you are struggling with weight, as are 65 percent of Americans, don't get discouraged and give up. You can succeed if you relearn how to eat. If I can do it, you can do it.

The Current High Profile Diets

Learning how to eat is considerably different than eating frozen prepared meals from Weight Watchers, Jenny Craig, or Nutrisystem. You can lose weight with all those programs and still never learn a thing about how to feed yourself healthy meals. The diet industry is huge. They make most of their money by selling you food supplements and prepared frozen meals, usually small portions with a low glycemic load—which is exactly what you need to learn how to do yourself. And sure, they'll give you the tasty sweets you see advertised on TV, because the portion served is the size of a quarter and the glycemic load is low. True, Weight Watchers and Jenny Craig will also weigh you and offer people-to-people support that can be helpful. The bottom line is unless you know how to control your own nutrition, invariably, either because of cost or lost interest, you'll drop out of these programs and gain the weight back.

Dr. Arthur Agatston's *South Beach Diet* is a low-carbohydrate diet, as is Atkins, but without Atkins' generosity of fats. (Atkins is discussed in Chapter 5.) Just for fun I logged on to the South Beach Diet website: www.SouthBeachDiet.com I submitted my weight, height, target weight, age, and gender and allowed them to give me my diet profile. According to them, my healthy weight is between 125-169 with an ideal BMI of between 18.2-25. Their data is straight from the published BMI charts, without recognition that the charts are unsuitable for an athletic person. I can't believe that they are actually suggesting that I could get down to a weight of 125 pounds and be healthy without a doctor ever seeing me. What a dangerous idea. If I ever got down to 125 I'd need nursing home care! The first phase of their diet program would be to totally give up all bread, rice, potatoes, pasta, baked goods, alcohol, and fruit for 14 days. After that, they bring some of the foods back, depending upon your progress.

As far as I can tell, South Beach doesn't sell foods, but they do push exercise equipment and other stuff. For $5 a week they'll also give you menus and advice. I question the advice to start with—you need carbohydrates from whole grains, fruits, and vegetables. My advice is to spend your $5 a week on buying healthy food. That said, Dr. Agatston is a highly respected cardiologist, and many people attest to being helped following his program. His books, which I haven't read, are also given high marks.

I've never tried Weight Watchers or the rest of the diets mentioned, but have tried diets taken from a couple of books. In 1985, as America and I were getting fatter following the low-fat, high-carb Western Diet, Harvey and Marilyn Diamond published a book titled, *Fit For Life*. The diet suggests that fruit be eaten, on its own, from the time one gets up until midday. Dinners are either a 'carbs meal' or a 'protein meal', and no combination of the two is permitted. The belief is that mixing protein and carbohydrates in the same meal prevents proper digestion and causes a build up of toxins, because the enzymes that digest protein cancel out the action of the enzymes that digest carbohydrates, and vice versa. All dairy products, and all products with refined sugar are forbidden.

As with other diets that heavily restrict food choices, many experts believe that the Fit For Life Diet doesn't provide proper nutrition. In the short run it does work though; I lost about 20 pounds before getting off it, and of course gained the weight back. It's a ridiculous diet on the face of it. For instance, I remember one evening at the old Airways Motel Restaurant in Buffalo New York, world renowned for their hot Buffalo wings, eating a platter of those tasty morsels dripping fat and not eating the carrots that came with them—just silly. You can still sign up for the "Fit For Life Weight Management System" at www.fitforlife.com

Dr. Barry Sears, a former researcher at the Boston University School of Medicine and the Massachusetts Institute of Technology, launched another weight loss/healthy eating diet program in 1995, with a very popular book titled, *The Zone*. His books have sold millions of copies. According to The Zone, achieving the right balance of carbohydrates, protein, and fats at every snack and meal creates the hormonal balance that will lead to weight loss, improved energy, and other health benefits. He claims you reach "the zone' by eating meals and snacks that contain precisely 9 grams of carbohydrate for every 7 grams of protein and 1.5 grams of fat. Pretty hard to calculate on the road, but here again he comes to the rescue with vitamin/mineral supplements, nutrition bars, and other foods. It's essentially a healthy diet that's hard to follow. I lost weight doing it for a while but gave up on it as being too complicated.

The perfectly balanced nutrition bars were very tasty, though. I found in taking one of them to the ski mountain for lunch, I'd most likely have a bowl of chili and eat it for desert. It's still a very active program that you can find at: www.zonediet.com Dr. Sears has gotten quite a lot of notoriety lately by helping really immense, bed-bound people lose hundreds of pounds.

The Zone did give me some good ideas that I incorporated in my successful 100-pound weight loss. So I didn't start clueless.

Without question, the best help I've found about eating right and weight control is The Healthy Eating Pyramid created by the faculty in the Department of Nutrition at the Harvard School of Public Health. I found Dr. Walter Willett, his book, *Eat, Drink, and Be Healthy,* and The Healthy Eating Pyramid while doing research for this book. You can do your research at: http://www.hsph.harvard.edu/nutritionsource/

While I'd already lost most of my weight before finding HSPH and The Healthy Eating Pyramid, it has helped tremendously in developing a long-term strategy of eating healthier. I relied heavily, and still do, on portion control and just about eliminated all bread and pasta from my diet. I knew nothing at all about the value of whole grains. Although I cut down on cheese, I still ate a fair amount, not realizing how high in saturated fat and calories it is. I thought cheese was high in protein and calcium, and therefore healthy. I've learned a tremendous amount from HSPH, including the values of various foods, food supplements, and the glycemic index and glycemic load to name a few.

Now I eat small portions of whole grains, including whole grain pasta, which has broadened my diet. I've cut way back on the cheese. I'm getting plenty of protein and calcium from other sources not packaged with saturated fat and high calories. As a result of understanding the science supporting The Healthy Eating Pyramid, I'm able to make better choices and to maintain a healthy weight quite easily.

One of the things I suggest is to think in terms of weekly menus. Families, by tradition, used to do that all the time. For example: fish on Friday (Catholics used to be prohibited from eating meat on Friday), pasta on Sunday, etc.—basically, recognizing that although you need daily nutrition, including carbohydrates, fats, and protein, you can and should vary the foods you get them from over a period of time. For instance, you might threat yourself to an ice cream every couple of weeks, but not daily.

We'll get to The Healthy Eating Pyramid, which I recommend, the original USDA's Food Pyramid and their current MyPyramid, the Mediterranean Pyramid, and other traditional food pyramids in Chapter 12.

Chapter 11

Two Martini Diet

While it may seem like it's a long time into the book to finally get down to what I actually eat, we couldn't discuss my meal choices intelligently until you had a handle on some of the science of nutrition, and were aware of the deadly risks of being overweight. I sure wish I had the information I've learned in researching this book long before now; I have struggled with the weight issue all my life. From the time I was a teenager, I always thought of myself as being fat, although I was never obese as many kids are today. I was just chubby and my self-image suffered for it. When I see the really obese kids around today my heart truly goes out to them as it's not only their health that's suffering, they're mentally paying a price as well. We live in a world of svelte TV images and bruised egos.

If you're thinking about imitating my success, here are twelve tips I've learned to get you started:

It's Not A Diet

Don't think of it as a diet, you're going to change the way you eat and live for the rest of your life.

Team Up

If you're married or have a life partner, do it together and support one another. Without that support it would be like trying to stop smoking with a smoker in the house—tough to do.

Goals

Set reasonable goals. If you can average a weight loss of a pound a week, you'd be doing great—that's 50 pounds in a year. My original goal was just that, to lose 50 pounds and get back down to 220 pounds. When I reached that goal at the end of a year, I'd found it so easy and comfortable that I just kept going down another 50 pound the following year (170 down from 270). Remember to lose a pound of fat a week requires burning 3,500 calories, 500 calories a day more than you're eating. I work on the reward system. The 500 calories I burn a day by exercise I reward with two martinis (about 300 calories); the rest of my weight loss was from changing my eating habits. Now I've stabilized my weight at just less than 170 pounds and have added more whole grains to my meals. My doctor and I agree that 170 pounds is a healthy weight for me. As this is written I've dropped down to 167 pounds—I've been doing a lot of spring-clean-up work outdoors, but I won't let it drop below 165 pounds.

Keep An Eye On Your BMR

Keep in mind that your basal metabolic rate (BMR) uses two-thirds to three-quarters of the calories burned each day. For a 165 pound person that's a calorie a minute, or 1440 calories a day, doing absolutely nothing but allowing your body to function. That gives you a major head start. After that, the more physical activity you do, the more calories you'll burn. I think most people who don't have a physically demanding job, like construction work, or being a rickshaw driver, need to deliberately exercise at least an hour a day to lose weight. Some of that can be by taking the stairs instead of the elevator, parking your car so that you have to walk, walking fast instead of sauntering, cutting your own grass instead of having the kid next door it. In short, just by being more physically active in your day-to-day life, instead of being a couch potato. (See Physical Activity and Exercise, Chapter 15.)

Plateaus

Expect plateaus. When you lose a lot of weight, your body goes through tremendous changes; it can take time for it to catch up. Don't get discouraged; first thing you know you'll miraculously drop two pounds overnight.

Snacks

If you get ravenous, eat a small low calorie snack, such as a carrot or piece of celery or a handful of nuts and/or drink a glass of water. The hunger will pass. You'll find as you eat less your stomach shrinks and is satisfied with less. As a general rule, though, don't eat between meals.

Don't Eat Where Your Car Does

Unlike years past, today there's almost no such thing as a gas station, they're all gas/junk food stations. Don't be tempted to buy a candy bar "for the road."

Take The Time To Sit At A Table

Eat sitting at a table, preferably with your family and/or friends, and preferably at regular meal times. Unfortunately, along with our obesity epidemic, many Americans are also working themselves to death. There are many tough choices in these tough economic times, but you need to be healthy to survive them.

Serve Meals, Not Help Yourself

Don't put everything you've cooked on the table and serve yourselves. Prepare the plates away from the table. Second portions are only for those who want to be the size of two people. Understandably, when you have guests for dinner it's a different situation. They should make their own choices as to whether or not to have seconds; nobody wants to be thought of as being stingy.

Small Plates, Small Portions

Use smaller plates. Vegetables should take up half the space on the plate—four-to-eight ounces of red meat, poultry, or fish don't take up that much room. Four ounces is about the size of a deck of cards. Spend a week using measuring cups and a food scale to get an accurate idea of what portion control really means. What do 4 or 8 ounces of meat, or a cup of vegetables, or a scoop of brown rice or other grain look like on your plate? Once you get the hang of it you won't have to continually measure. It isn't rocket science. I have a digital scale put out by Escali; it works great for weighing both food and also mail for correct postage.

Stop Eating When Satisfied

Don't ever force yourself to finish everything on your plate. If you feel satisfied, stop eating. My wife and I often will serve an eight-ounce serving of red meat, poultry, or fish and save three ounces for part of lunch the next day. If you're worried about waste, think about which costs more, medical bills or perhaps a few ounces of lost food? With two large Airedales, we rarely have that problem in any case. But don't use your pets as disposals; it's not healthy for them to be fat either.

Eat Slowly

Eat slowly and enjoy. Food is one of the great pleasures of life. We'll talk more about alcohol use later, but one of the advantages of having a drink or two with dinner is to help us slow down and relax. It would be a rare Italian or French meal that didn't have wine on the table. In Germany it might be some of their excellent beer. And guess what? Their rate of obesity is nowhere near as high as ours, although it's a growing problem in other countries as people get hooked on our Western Diet. I don't think there's a major city in the world that doesn't have a McDonald's. Heck, there's one at the foot of the Spanish Steps in Rome, which serves wine, incidentally.

Recipes and Menus

Believe me, in all that I've written during my life I never once contemplated writing about food recipes and menus. There are hundreds, if not thousands, of cookbooks written by world-renowned chefs and I'm certainly not one of them. We have a couple hundred cookbooks ourselves, most of which I've never read, but my wife Sue does. You should have a couple of good ones as well. It will help you to think in terms of small gourmet meals rather than large ranch-hand size ones. There's a great section in *Eat, Drink, and Be Healthy* devoted only to recipes. What follows is merely an effort to share with you typical meals that have enabled me to lose weight and maintain a healthy weight.

As said before, my initial approach was, and remains, portion control, and cutting way back on highly processed white bread, pasta, and potatoes. I didn't learn about the benefits of substituting whole grains until I lost most of my weight. That came later with *Eat, Drink, and Be Healthy*. Sugared drinks and junk foods, such as potato chips and candy, I simply eliminated. Otherwise, unknowingly, we were pretty much in step with Dr. Willett's recommendations and the Healthy Eating Pyramid.

Here are some sample meals and recipes:

Pre-Breakfast

I'm an early riser, usually up shaved and showered by 7:00 A.M. I enjoy my first cup of black, leftover coffee while brewing a new pot, grab a banana or other piece of fruit, some dog biscuits for Spencer and Tracy, our two Airedales, and head down to my office, where I'll usually work until 8:30 or 9:00.

Breakfast

A second cup of coffee, which I rarely finish, often a small cup of low-fat yogurt with fruit or a small cup of low-fat cottage cheese, sometimes a slice of cantaloupe, which our Bengal cat Tiger loves to share with me (his relatives, generations removed, were Asian Leopard Cats); and then the main course, which I rotate between a toasted slice of whole-grain bread with either peanut butter or low-fat cream cheese, or a small bowl of whole-grain cereal, either hot or cold, with skim milk. This morning just for chuckles, my second fruit and main course was a tomato salad with a few slices of fresh, hard-crusted, dense Italian bread. The dressing I used can be used anytime as a bread dip substitute for butter. It's very simple to make; we learned it from our friend Karen Robert. Here's her recipe that will serve four as a dip:

Ingredients—extra virgin olive oil, finely chopped sun-dried tomato, a little
Italian seasoning, garlic, balsamic vinegar and sea salt. For proportions:

1 cup of extra virgin olive oil
1 Tbs. finely chopped sun-dried tomato,
1 Tbs. dried Italian seasoning
1 or 2 lg. clove(s) of garlic (more or less according to how strong you like the garlic flavor)
1/2 to 1 tsp. sea salt (more or less to taste, but don't leave out completely)
1 Tbs. balsamic vinegar

Slightly crush the garlic clove and mix it into the rest of the ingredients. Best if made at least a few hours before serving so that flavors blend together. Can be kept in a covered glass or stainless steel container for up to a week.

Tips: Eat the fruit, don't substitute juice, which is likely to have three times as many calories and little of the fiber, and avoid breakfast meats. They're high in saturated fat and calories and a good way to wreck your diet for the day.

Sunday Brunch

We call it going to church. Sue and I have being doing Sunday brunch at Lloyd Hills Restaurant in the adjoining town of Bethlehem for many years. It's great. While Mother lived with us she loved it. We usually bring a guest or two and look forward to seeing the regulars and the owners and staff.

Sue usually starts out with a glass of wine, I with either a glass of wine or a tall Tanqueray Gin bloody Mary, with a large stalk of celery. My usual starter course is a small crock of union soup with a topping of mozzarella cheese. (I can always plan on Sue stealing some.) Last Sunday for my main course I had three soft poached eggs on 7-grain whole grain toast, no meat, and no potatoes, with a small salad on the side sprinkled with walnuts, olive oil, and wine vinegar. The owners, Dianna and Bill Greene, are threatening to put some of my breakfasts on the menu as Jerry's specials. Note that unless bread is fresh baked with a hard crust I always toast it, which lowers the glycemic load. Also, Sunday brunch comes only once a week, and even though we eat a light dinner on Sunday night, I routinely gain a pound that it takes until Tuesday to lose.

Lunch

I find that if I don't eat by noon I start to get a little shaky. My body is ready for food. One of the tricks I've learned is to start with a low-calorie cup of soup; it helps you to feel full on less. I often use dried Lipton Chicken Soup; other times half a can of the various multi-bean soups that are out there. While the Lipton product only contains 40 calories, it is high on salt, so if that's a factor for you because of high blood pressure don't go there. Two cold soup summer treats are Borscht, a Russian, Ukrainian, and Yiddish soup made from red beets, and Gazpacho, a Spanish vegetable soup made from tomatoes, cucumbers, green peppers, olive oil, unions and garlic.

If I have leftover meat, fish, or veggies I'll nuke them and eat those or add to them for lunch. You'll be surprised. Just a few ounces of meat or fish can be very satisfying. I rarely eat sandwiches (two pieces of bread) anymore—too many calories. Other frequent choices are a small can of tuna fish, or sardines in olive oil, or herring in wine sauce (Nathan's brand), or a few pieces of sliced deli turkey. I'll add a piece of whole-grain toast or 4 or 5 Triscuits, which are whole grain wheat crackers put out by Nabisco. For a light sandwich, try using a small whole-grain pita. Add to this some carrots, celery, artichoke hearts, or a piece of cucumber and it's a nice meal of just a few hundred calories.

Another lunch I like is hummus on an unleavened matzo. Hummus is a popular Middle Eastern food made from chickpeas and matzo is a traditional Jewish large (7 X 6"), crispy, thin wafer (125 calories each). It's a delicious combination, which we often have with a few Italian sweet red peppers that have been bottled in olive oil. Hummus is now popular in supermarkets and produced in various flavors. So is matzo if you live anywhere near a Jewish community. We use Yehuda Matzos imported from Israel; they're very inexpensive and extra crisp.

Tips: When you eat lunch in a restaurant, ask what comes with the meal—many times it will be French Fries or potato chips. Tell your server you don't want them on your plate and they'll often offer coleslaw or sliced tomatoes in its place. I try to stick with salads but a sandwich can be okay if its on whole-grain bread. Remember, "club sandwiches" have three slices of bread. And stay out of the fast food palaces. There's nothing there you want, only some things that are worse than others. Remember, restaurants don't have to list trans fats and fast foods are loaded with both trans fats and saturated fat, to say nothing of sugar and salt.

Dinner

Here there's a lot more variety than breakfast and lunch, which tend to be rather routine. Dinner is a special time for us to be together, have a drink and celebrate our food. I certainly don't ever expect to be "fed" by Sue; it's strictly a joint enterprise with both of us selecting and preparing the meal, although she's our primary hunter/gatherer at the supermarket.

About shopping: What's your top priority in selecting the food you buy; is it quality or price? If it's the former you're making the right choice; the difference in price is probably less than 10 percent. Also when you're using smaller portions you're going to spend less anyway. With red meat and poultry the bargain packages are usually loaded with untrimmed fat buried on the bottom where you can't see it. You'll also get higher quality foods from a farmer's market or food co-op, both of which support local farmers, who as a rule grow crops with less commercial fertilizer and pesticides, and sometimes even meet the criteria to be labeled as grown organically. These products are more likely to contain the phytochemicals, vitamins, and other nutrients that your body needs than those grown on huge mono-crop commercial farms.

"Eat plenty of fruits and vegetables" is timeless advice that your mother probably gave you and that science is just recently catching up to. Since 1991, the experts have been recommending that we eat five servings of fruits and vegetables a day. The Harvard School of Public Health recommends eating no less than five servings a day and that you'll benefit even more from nine servings a day. HSPH also recommends that you vary which ones you eat. If you stroll down the produce department of a modern supermarket, you'll find about a hundred different kinds of fruits and vegetable of all colors to choose from. Of all the wonderful and nutritious options available, unbelievably, the average American relies on only twelve. And of these, their daily choices might be two glasses of orange juice, an apple, French fries at lunch, and a potato at dinner—hardly healthy but that meets the criteria established by the Dietary Guidelines for Americans, which, incidentally are the guidelines used by school cafeterias and other public institutions. In practice, a national survey showed that fewer than one in three Americans get five servings of fruits and vegetables a day.

So, clearly, if you want to get to and maintain a healthy weight, your goal should be to eat as many as nine servings a day of fruits and vegetables. And don't include white potatoes. I eat white potatoes very rarely, and have mostly eliminated them from my meals along with white bread, pasta, and rice.

Many vegetables can be eaten raw and are often used in salads; others taste better and are more palatable cooked to break down the fiber. Cold or cooked, both fruits and vegetables are also a good way to get your daily amount of the good fats by using olive and other vegetable oils in cooking or in salad dressings. The same is true for nuts—we often sprinkle walnuts, almonds, or pine nuts on salad. We also use fruit in salads a great deal. Everyone uses tomatoes and cucumbers, which are fruits (they have seeds). Add to your repertoire avocadoes, apples, grapes, and pears; they're delicious in leafy green salads. When you start combining fruits and vegetables into meals, it's really not that difficult to meet your goal of nine healthy and satisfying servings a day. It doesn't have to be huge amounts to count. Here's an orange salad recipe from Olive Nation as an example:

Sicilian Orange Salad

Ingredients are 4 juicy oranges, salt and freshly ground black pepper, 10 black olives, pitted and cut in half, 1 small white onion thinly sliced, 4 tbsp extra virgin olive oil.

Peel the oranges, taking care to remove all the white pith. Slice thinly and place in a salad bowl. Sprinkle with a little salt, than add olives and onion. Drizzle with the oil and season with a generous grinding of pepper.

A light, dry white wine goes well with it.

Now that you're embarking on a new way of eating that makes fruits and vegetable the centerpiece of most meals, here are a few ideas for dinners we like that fit into the program very nicely. The first few require a fair degree of preparation and cooking time so we don't have them often. I'll make it when we have guests or infrequently, if it's just the two of us, we'll have a few meals then freeze the rest. Alternately of course you can make a smaller batch.

Mother's Escarole Soup

Rare was the meal that mother didn't serve a cooked green vegetable and escarole soup was and remains one of my favorites, although over time I've added to her recipe. I use a five-quart pot with a lid.

The ingredients are 3 large heads of fresh escarole (we also substitute broccoli raab, or kale for a different flavor), a large white onion, fresh garlic, a large can of cannellini beans (we also use chick peas or black beans), a frozen package of cheese tortellini, salt, black and red pepper, a large box of low fat chicken broth, and olive oil.
Preparation

Separate the escarole leaves from the heads breaking the larger outside ones in two and wash in a sink full of cold water—when rinsed clean pile them on a drain board.

Skin and cut the onion into quarters and then those into ¼" slices that break apart. Put the onions into the pot in a nice float of olive oil and season with salt, black pepper, and just a little hot red pepper – enough to give the soup a bite. Next open several large cloves of garlic (we like a lot), and dice the garlic. Open the box of chicken broth and put it aside. Over a medium hot burner sweat the onions until they're beginning to brown, then add the garlic (garlic takes much less time to brown). Now add the whole box of broth.

When the pot begins to bubble start adding the escarole, it will seem to fill the pot but it boils down quickly and you'll have no trouble getting in the 3 heads. At this point you'll have to add water to fill the pot to an inch or an inch and a half below the top. Turn the burner on low, cover the pot with the lid cracked so the pot can vent a little, and let cook a hour or so.

Next strain and add the cannellini beans and stir in. Check the fluid level, recover and let cook for another hour or so. Then turn the pot off.

An hour or so before you're ready to eat bring the pot back up to a bubble and add the frozen tortellini, it will take about 20 minutes at a low bubble to cook. Turn the pot off and let the brew "settle." It's best served hot, but not steaming hot, in a bowl. A piece of fresh-baked whole-grain bread on the side for dunking probably won't break your calorie bank.

The whole pot can serve a lot of people, so it's great for guests and a dish most people have never had. A glass or two of red zinfandel goes really well with the meal, as does a little fruit and a small cup of Italian expresso coffee for dessert.

Jerry's Famous Chicken Soup

If you think you're getting a cold, this is the cure, and I feel comfortable saying that without anything that remotely resembling a license to practice medicine. What all the mothers and grandmothers, whether Italian or Jewish, have said through the years is true, there's nothing better than chicken soup to chase away a cold.

The ingredients are 4 whole chicken legs (thighs & drumstick – I separate them), a box of low-fat chicken broth, carrots, parsnips, celery, white onions, parsley, dill, salt and black pepper.

Preparation

Again use the 5-quart pot and lid.

Wash the chicken legs and trim all the lose fat. Add the broth and water to the pot with enough fluid to cover the legs but not too fill, there's a lot of stuff to add; season with salt and lots of black pepper.

Skin and slice 1 and 1/2 onions (don't dice them, this is a hearty soup) and add to the pot.

Using a 1-quart measuring cup, fill it about two-thirds with chopped carrots, pieces about a half-inch thick. Add it to the soup and stir it in. Repeat the process with equal amounts of celery and parsnips – good bite size pieces.

Chop and add a good fat bunch of parsley and stir in.

Last, chop two packages of fresh dill – the way it's sold one package isn't enough. Add and stir in. This gives the soup a very distinctive taste.

The pot can now be filled with water to just below the top, the burner turned low to simmer and cover with a cracked lid. Allow the soup to cook very slowly for about two hours, checking the fluid level ever half hour or so. When done, allow the soup to "settle" for a half hour before serving. It should be served hot but not steaming hot.

Now you have a choice to make. What kind of whole-grain carbohydrate do you want to serve in the soup? It could be whole-wheat small pasta elbows, or whole-wheat or corn spaghetti broken into fist-size pieces, or brown rice—they're all good. Cook them in a separate pot, drain and add to the bowls when served. The portion of grain should be about 2 ounces per bowl.

Here again this can easily serve six people with some left over.

Eggplant Lasagna

We've all had lasagna made with wide pasta noodles, layered with ricotta cheese, mozzarella cheese, tomato sauce, and sometime s ground beef. It can also be done with layers of sliced & pressed eggplant and a few layers of whole-wheat lasagna pasta, sans ground beef – it's great, and a healthier combination with a lower glycemic load. A little low-fat ricotta and mozzarella won't kill you either. Think of this as a special treat that you won't eat very often.

The ingredients are whole-wheat lasagna pasta (I get them online from Barry Farm Foods – through Amazon.com), tomato sauce (we us Classico, Tomato & Basil and add a can of fresh whole tomatoes, olive oil, garlic), 3 eggplants (the smaller ones are most tender), low-fat (skim milk) ricotta cheese, low-fat mozzarella, Italian breadcrumbs, an egg, and grated Parmesan cheese. _

Use a disposable aluminum oven lasagna pan, they're cheap, deep, and not worth the effort of cleaning.

Pre-cook the lasagna pasta in water with a little olive oil and salt – the oil prevents the pasta from sticking and makes it easier to separate. Only partially cook, it will finish cooking in the oven with the lasagna.

Cut the eggplants with skin on crossways relatively thin, about ¼". Stack the slices in an oven pan with toweling between layers, cover with another pan and weight it with a few heavy cans letting the water leach out for about an hour or so.

Prepare your tomato sauce in a deep frying pan by browning some garlic (to taste – we like a lot) in olive oil, and then add the Classico and fresh tomato. Cook slowly until the fresh tomatoes are broken down.

Dice the mozzarella, and separately blend the ricotta in a mixing bowl with a beaten egg and some Italian breadcrumbs.

Now build your lasagna in layers, first some sauce on the bottom of the pan, then a layer of pasta laid length wise, then a layer of eggplant. Drizzle some sauce and add some diced mozzarella and some of the ricotta mix. Repeat the process only this time lay the pasta crosswise. You may get two or three layers of each but don't fill to the pan to very top or it will bubble over and make a mess. The top layer should be sauce, topped with some additional breadcrumbs and grated Parmesan cheese.

It will take about 45 minutes to cook in a pre-heated 350-degree oven. When it starts to bubble on top it's done. It needs to cool for a half hour or it will be tough to cut into serving portions.

A pan has a lot of serving but don't feel compelled to eat them all! Cut into individual portions; it freezes well and is good for a handful of meals.

Although this meal is tasty and loaded with good stuff, it lacks something green. Serve it with a green leafy salad on the side. The same is true any of the red sauce pasta meals. We use the same sauce with either whole wheat or corn spaghetti or macaroni. You may have trouble getting corn pastas at a supermarket—the price has shot up because corn is being diverted into ethanol rather than food. It's more profitable. I just order a batch on line from OliveNation at: www.olivenation.com

I like a nice fruity merlot with red sauce, but good imported Italian Chianti also works.

Pasta & Broccoli

I learned this one at an Italian restaurant in Wiesbaden, Germany; they had it on the menu, and cooked it quickly to order. It's a stovetop dinner that's simple and fast to make.

The ingredients are fresh broccoli, one of the whole-grain pastas (I like fist size broken spaghetti), chick peas, olive oil, onion and garlic, salt and black and red pepper.

Use a deep large frying pan, the same kind you'd use for red tomato sauce.

Break a head of broccoli into small flowerets; you can cut the stems into small pieces as well. Rinse and drain. Remember, your goal is 2 ounces of dry pasta for each serving—that's not a lot but it can be extremely satisfying and enough. Use the food scale until you can eyeball it.

Start by browning sliced onion and the broccoli in a generous amount of olive oil. When almost done add the garlic (it burns easily). Then add hot water (be careful it doesn't spatter on you) and bring to a bubble, add drained chick peas and the pasta, cover and cook on medium low heat until the pasta is cooked. You may have to add water as the pasta absorbs it. I like it kind of soupy rather than soggy.

Sue's Pesto

This is another pasta dinner that's fast and easy to make.

Ingredients are an amount dependant on number of servings of your whole-grain pasta of choice (for this one I prefer the corn), 3 cups washed and dried coarsely chopped fresh basil, 1 tablespoon parsley, 2-3 tablespoons pine nuts (or walnuts), 4 cloves garlic, 1 & ½ cups extra virgin olive oil, 1/8 teaspoon nutmeg, 8 oz. grated Parmesan cheese, and salt and black pepper. Use low-fat chicken broth for thinning.

For this, cook the pasta separately as directed in boiling water.

Process the ingredients in a food processor until smooth to your taste.

Serve in bowls with some of the pesto poured on top – not too much, you can always add more. This recipe is enough to go with about a pound of pasta but properly covered it can be refrigerated for some time, or even frozen in ice cube trays that will stay almost indefinitely.

A green leafy salad with avocado goes with it nicely.

Meat, Poultry & Fish

As a rule we'll have a fish and vegetarian dinner at least once a week. The rest we'll alternate with meals having small portions of beef, veal, pork, lamb, chicken, and turkey. The major portions of these meals will be cooked vegetables, salads, fruits, and occasionally a sweet potato or brown rice. We eat most of our whole-grains at breakfast and lunch.

I don't have any special recipes but I can give you some helpful tips:

- We like our steak cooked medium rare over a char-grill. The only cut of beef that is cut small (8 oz. or less) and thick enough to cook well over a grill is filet mignon, which is expensive. We do that sometimes but alternatively we'll buy a thick cut, of lean, Delmonico or New York strip steak weighing about a pound and cut it in half. Also, to cut down on saturated fats always buy lean cuts of beef and low-percentage fat ground beef (90 percent lean). Trim any edge fat that remains on the steaks.

- You can usually find 8 oz. or less cut veal, pork, or lamb chops. We usually cook these in a little olive oil in a well-seasoned heavy cast iron frying pan with a cover. Since these are staples you can same money by buying them in bulk when on sale, dividing them into serving portions and freezing.

♦ When it comes to poultry don't forget turkey. Sliced turkey breast is lean and makes terrific turkey cutlets. I make them the same way I do chicken cutlets. This one I'll share with you: All you need is the sliced breasts (not cut too thick), Italian breadcrumbs, and a couple of eggs. The German/Austrian version is called schnitzel, originally made with thin sliced veal and called Wiener schnitzel. It's also made with thin cut pork. I had both often in Germany.

I usually beat two whole eggs in a bowl, but if you have a cholesterol problem beat just the egg whites. Put the breadcrumbs in another bowl or deep dish. First dip the cutlets fully coating them in the egg and then dip them in the breadcrumbs, completely covering them. Transfer to a platter. I usually make enough for two meals; they're great served either hot or cold.

I quick fry them in a 50/50 mixture of olive oil and vegetable oil using a medium high heat that's a little too hot for straight olive oil. You have to really stand over them while cooking as they take very little time. When the edges first start to turn brown turn them over. Don't overcook. Line a clean serving platter with paper towels to absorb excess oil.

The leftover egg and breadcrumbs can be mixed together and quickly cooked in the leftover oil to make a frittata (a Spanish omelet). We use that as a treat for the Airedales, although we snitch some too.

I usually serve the cutlets with a tomato salad with basil, onion, and olive oil and wine vinegar.

♦ We rarely eat sausages, chicken livers, and calf's liver, although it's a treat on occasion. Baked ham (the thigh and rump of pork) is sometimes a holiday treat to be shared with guests, as whole turkeys, legs of lamb, or large cuts of roast beef. Once again, think of portion control, not deprivation. Such foods are some of life's treats.

♦ Rule number one when it comes to fish is, if you overcook it you ruin it. If the fish is fresh or was fresh frozen you can eat it raw as sushi. If it isn't you shouldn't eat anyway, so don't kill it by overcooking. We eat a wide variety of fish. Some fresh ocean blue fish and striped bass, which I used to catch, are now hard to come by, but others such as salmon, trout, catfish, tilapia, halibut, tuna, cod, haddock, herring, mackerel, monkfish, red snapper, flounder, sea-trout, swordfish, and tilefish are still available, at least for awhile, until our lack of worldwide conservation makes them a thing of the past. When you add to this list lobster, shrimp, Alaskan king crab legs, clams, oysters, and God knows what else, there's no reason to miss out on diet rich in sea foods, and one or two meals a week will not expose you to enough mercury to be problematic.

The fragile flaky fish we'll lightly batter with flour and pan-fry, the others we'll usually cook in the oven with a simple lemon, wine, butter/olive oil dressing.

The challenge with your common everyday meals is to eat variety of foods. The truth is at this point science doesn't know everything your body needs for good health. Accordingly, your safest bet is get the basic food groups every day and a great variety of foods over time. Portion control and eliminating the garbage gives you a lot of leeway to experiment—and it doesn't have to be perfect, nobody or anything is.

Spices and flavors are important to small portion gourmet style meals. Use the newly purchased cookbooks I've suggested that you buy for ideas and get a small chest of spices. They're not expensive and they last forever. There are a number of excellent oil and vinegar choices. Olive, corn, and other vegetable oils should be stables, but also try walnut, hazelnut, and almond oils. They'll give different and distinctive flavors to your salads and veggies. The same with vinegar.

While red wine vinegar is good for a lot of things, there are others that add distinctive flavors, such as Balsamic, rice, fig, and tarragon vinegars. Balsamic vinegar over fresh strawberries sweetens them like sugar.

Break the mold, get wild and crazy and try vegetables you haven't used before. I mentioned some in the recipes. Here are others that we like: whole artichokes, beets, bok choy, Brussels sprouts, cabbage, chard, cauliflower, fresh corn, endive, mint, peas, peppers, radishes, squash, sweet potatoes, and turnips.

Chapter 12

Food Pyramids

Food pyramids are graphic depictions of diets that simply direct you to eat more of the foods at the bottom and less of the ones at the top. In this chapter we'll focus on the first USDA Food Guide Pyramid (1992-2005), the revised USDA MyPyramid.gov (2005), and the Department of Nutrition - Harvard School of Public Health's Healthy Eating Pyramid, published in Dr. Willett's *Eat, Drink and Be Healthy* (1st edition 2001, 2nd 2005). We'll also look at four traditional diets representing different cultures presented by the Oldways Preservation & Exchange Trust. Oldways is a widely respected nonprofit food issues think tank located in Boston. The four diets are: Mediterranean, Asian, Latin American, and vegetarian.

First let's look at the role of the United States government in all this. The United States Department of Agriculture (USDA), and the Department of Health and Human Services (HHS) have jointly published the *Dietary Guidelines for Americans*, as required by law every five years since 1980. You can access the Guidelines website at: health.gov/DietaryGuideline. According to the USDA and HHS, the "The Guidelines provide authoritative advice for people two years and older about how good dietary habits can promote health and reduce risk for major chronic diseases. They serve as the basis for Federal food and nutrition education programs." The 2005 Guidelines is an 84-

page document available by navigating their website. The next Dietary Guidelines for Americans is scheduled to be published in 2010. The makeup of that Dietary Guidelines Advisory Committee (DGAC) to accomplish that should be announced sometime in 2008.

Let's pause and examine the HHS and USDA self-phrased mission statement for the Guidelines, first to "provide authoritative advice…" Sounds good but how many Americans actually read them? I never did until doing this research; all I knew of the 1992-2005 Guidelines was the food pyramid graphic, which was taught in schools, and appeared on cereal boxes and food labels; many doctor's offices had them plastered on a wall. You can find the 1992 Guidelines (as amended in 1995) at: nal.usda.gov/fnic/dga/dguide95.html. As for the 2005 edition, I'm confident that not too many of us have or will read that 84-page tome. The only way you can find MyPyramid is online. It's an interactive program with more color than substance. It's not available in print and is, incidentally, no longer a traditional food pyramid, which made it is easier to understand. The second part of the mission statement is where the big money comes in; "They [the Guidelines] serve as the basis for federal food and nutrition education programs." Those Federal programs set the standards for food stamps, school lunch programs, and food services for the armed forces and federal prisons. Combined with swaying public opinion as to food choices there are billions of dollars on the table in a high-stakes political poker game as to what the Guidelines recommend. It's the reason Burger King and Pizza Hut are readily available at military bases all over the world, even in Iraq, catered by Halliburton.

Here is how Dr. Willett portrays how the Guidelines are contrived; "It supposed to be a scholarly and scientific process, but is often a free-for-all among lobbyists for agribusiness, food companies, and special interest groups."

In President George W. Bush's administration, under-the-table deals were routinely cut with big business and sound public policy often played second fiddle to cronyism. You can read more about that in another of my books, *Facing Fascism, The Threat to American Democracy in the 21st Century*. A prime example I focused on was an energy bill secretly crafted in Vice President Cheney's back room in collusion with the big oil and coal producers and costing the taxpayers billions. The responsibility for producing the 2005 Guidelines fell to Secretaries Ann M. Veneman (USDA) and Tommy G. Thomson (HHS), with much the same outcome as the energy bill: agribusiness, food companies, and special interests, were able to protect their highly profitable junk foods at the risk of the public's health. It started with the bizarre appointment of Dr. Eric Hentges as executive director of the Center for Nutritional Policy and Promotion (CNPP) in February 2003 (he served until November 2007). The CNPP oversees the planning, development and review of the Guidelines as a subdivision of the USDA. Dr. Hentges was an expert in animal nutrition—not human nutrition—whose previous jobs had been with the National Livestock and Meat Board, the National Pork Producers Association, and the National Pork Board.

The thirteen members of Dietary Guidelines Advisory Committee who worked on the 2005 Guidelines were human nutrition experts from Johns Hopkins, Harvard, Penn State, and Columbia, to name a few of the prestigious universities that they hailed from, who, apparently from all that I've read, produced a high-quality technical report. However, that committee was instructed to turn the report over to a second committee to be translated into useful Guidelines. The second committee was never formed and the Guidelines were written in obscurity by those held unaccountable. The USDA then contracted with the public relations giant Porter-Novelli to design MyPyramid, its Web site, and the marketing program to promote it. The company certainly knows how to sell junk foods; its other clients, current or former, included McDonald's, Krispy Kreme, Johnnie Walker, and Masterfoods USA, whose products include Wrigley chewing gums, Mars Bars, M&M's, Twix, Skittles, and Snickers.

When Secretaries Ann M. Veneman (USDA), a former food-industry lobbyist, and Tommy G. Thomson (HHS), a former governor of Wisconsin, announced the new Dietary Guidelines for Americans at a press conference on January 12, 2005, they were bombarded with questions regarding transparent faults concerning the lack of warnings against trans fats, sugars, salt, and rapidly digested carbohydrates. At the end of the conference Secretary Thomson summarized by saying, "... the truth of the matter is, it's up to the individual. You're going to have to watch what you eat, and you're going to have to exercise. That's what the report says." Essentially, he confirmed that the lobbyists had held their ground and the administration wasn't about to buck them. As a result, now we're advised that all foods can be part of a healthy and balanced diet and that there is no such thing as a bad food; it's all about personal responsibility. Apparently the USDA and HHS accept none of their responsibility to protect us or help us make those wise choices. And Americans keep getting fatter and more and more of us suffer from chronic diseases. We'll focus on MyPyramid a little later. First, the original 1992 Food Guide Pyramid.

The USDA's Original

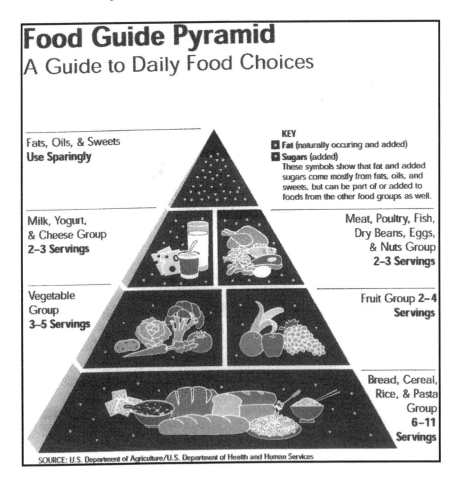

Food Guide Pyramid
A Guide to Daily Food Choices

Fats, Oils, & Sweets
Use Sparingly

KEY
■ Fat (naturally occuring and added)
▼ Sugars (added)
These symbols show that fat and added sugars come mostly from fats, oils, and sweets, but can be part of or added to foods from the other food groups as well.

Milk, Yogurt,
& Cheese Group
2–3 Servings

Meat, Poultry, Fish,
Dry Beans, Eggs,
& Nuts Group
2–3 Servings

Vegetable
Group
3–5 Servings

Fruit Group 2–4
Servings

Bread, Cereal,
Rice, & Pasta
Group
**6–11
Servings**

SOURCE: U.S. Department of Agriculture/U.S. Department of Health and Human Services

According to Dr. Willett and his associates at the Harvard School of Public Health, this 1992 food pyramid was ill-advised from the start and well out of date when he and his associates published their own Healthy Eating Pyramid in 2001. They not only had the advantage of a lot more scientific information than the USDA had in 1992; they also didn't have to negotiate with special interests. He lays out the Food Guide Pyramid's six most health-damaging faults. We've already discussed the reasons why they are faults in our study of nutrients. Here is a recap:

1. *Al fats are bad.* Wrong—some fats are good for you.
2. *All carbohydrates are good.* Wrong again—some are, some aren't.
3. *Protein sources are interchangeable.* Not true—some sources of protein are better for you than others.
4. *Dairy products are essential.* Not true—you can get plenty of calcium from other sources that are not high in saturated fat and calories.
5. *Eat your potatoes.* Not true—white potatoes have a high glycemic load and a lot of calories.
6. *No guidance on weight, exercise, alcohol, and vitamins.* The Food Guide Pyramid is silent on all these issues.

Other obvious faults to me as a layperson are that the Guidelines pyramid graphic recommends 6-11 servings of grain. It's only if you read the text that you learn that 11 servings are only appropriate for those needing a very high caloric diet. Also, the graphic speaks of servings that are only defined in the text—what is a serving? For red meat, fish and poultry, a serving is 2-3 ounces, which is unrealistically low. On the other hand, 11 servings of grain a day, by their measure, could be a gut-busting pound or more of white bread, pasta, and cereal, which have an enormously high glycemic load.

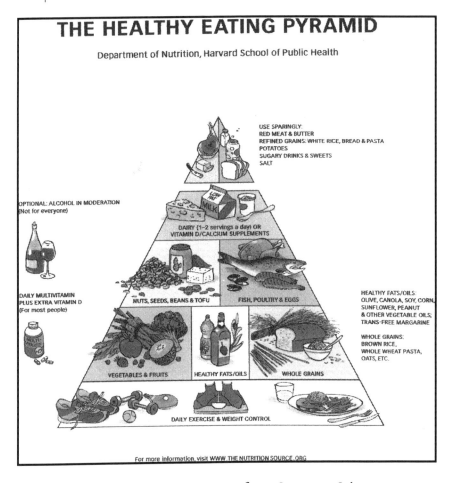

THE HEALTHY EATING PYRAMID

Department of Nutrition, Harvard School of Public Health

USE SPARINGLY:
RED MEAT & BUTTER
REFINED GRAINS: WHITE RICE, BREAD & PASTA
POTATOES
SUGARY DRINKS & SWEETS
SALT

OPTIONAL: ALCOHOL IN MODERATION
(Not for everyone)

DAIRY (1–2 servings a day) OR
VITAMIN D/CALCIUM SUPPLEMENTS

DAILY MULTIVITAMIN
PLUS EXTRA VITAMIN D
(For most people)

HEALTHY FATS/OILS:
OLIVE, CANOLA, SOY, CORN,
SUNFLOWER, PEANUT
& OTHER VEGETABLE OILS;
TRANS-FREE MARGARINE

WHOLE GRAINS:
BROWN RICE,
WHOLE WHEAT PASTA,
OATS, ETC.

NUTS, SEEDS, BEANS & TOFU   FISH, POULTRY & EGGS

VEGETABLES & FRUITS   HEALTHY FATS/OILS   WHOLE GRAINS

DAILY EXERCISE & WEIGHT CONTROL

For more information, visit WWW.THE NUTRITION SOURCE.ORG

Reproduced with permission from Simon & Schuster

As said earlier, the Healthy Eating Pyramid was built by Dr. Willett and his associates at Harvard to offer sound scientific guidance to people in the face of faulted recommendations by the USDA and the HHS nearly a decade before. It was included in the first edition of *Eat, Drink, and Be Healthy*, first published in 2001. The second edition, published in 2005, points out the faults in MyPyramid as well. What you see above is the 2008-updated version of The Healthy Eating Pyramid. The book is readily available at bookstores and the Healthy Eating Pyramid and narrative can be found online at: http://www.hsph.harvard.edu/nutritionsource/what-should-you-eat/pyramid/index.html

In the way of a brief bio, Dr. Walter Willett went to medical school at the University of Michigan, and then did his internship and residency in internal medicine at the Harvard Medical Service of Boston City Hospital. And, as he puts it, "While this experience was very rewarding…I came to realize that the typical problems of our patients, such as heart disease, diabetes, and cancer, were seldom cured and often unsatisfactorily managed."

Wanting to understand the root causes and potential prevention of these conditions, he went back to school and achieved a doctorial degree in epidemiology at Harvard School of Public Health. He is now Chairman of the Department of Nutrition at HSPH and Professor of Medicine at Harvard Medical School.

Since the late 1970s, Dr. Willett has focused much of his work on developing both questionnaires and biochemical approaches to study the effects of diet on the occurrence of major diseases in large populations. He began by working on the Nurses Health Study, which was established by Dr. Frank Speizer in 1976 with funding from the National Institute of Health. This involved a base of approximately 122,000 nurses. In 1980 they sent out the first dietary questionnaire to participants and have been continually updating the information ever since. In 1986 they added 52,000 men via the Health Professionals' Follow-up Study, and in 1989 Dr. Willett and colleagues developed the Nurses Health Study II that added another 116,000 women. Every two years, cohort members receive a follow-up questionnaire with questions about diseases and health-related topics, including smoking, hormone use, pregnancy history, and menopausal status. They're now working on establishing Nurses Health Study III. You can learn more about the Nurses' Health Study online at: (http://www.channing.harvard.edu/nhs/); you may wish to participate.

All together the Healthy Eating Pyramid is built upon the latest nutritional science and the accumulated diet-related health data of a population of about 300,000 people. Brick by brick, from the website, here's how the pyramid is built from the bottom up:

Exercise and Weight Control

The Healthy Eating Diet sits on a foundation of daily exercise and weight control because these two related elements have the strongest influence on your chances of staying healthy. It's back to the simple rule of energy balance: Weight change = calories in − calories out. If you burn as many calories as you take in each day, there's nothing left over for storage in fat cells, and weight remains the same. Eat more than you burn and you end up adding fat and pounds. Eat less and you'll lose weight. Regular daily exercise is essential to control your weight, and is a key part in any weight-loss effort.

Whole Grains

The body needs carbohydrates mainly for energy. The best sources of carbohydrates are whole grains such as oatmeal, whole wheat bread, and brown rice. They deliver the outer (bran) and inner (germ) layers along with energy-rich starch. The body can't digest whole grains as quickly as it can highly processed carbohydrates such as white flour. This keeps blood sugar and insulin levels from rising, then falling, too quickly. Better control of blood sugar and insulin can keep hunger at bay and may prevent the development of type 2 diabetes. Plus, a growing body of research suggests that eating a diet rich in whole grains may also protect against heart disease.

Healthy Fats and Oils

Surprised that the Healthy Eating Pyramid puts some fats near the base, indicating they are okay to eat? Although this recommendation seems to go against conventional wisdom, it's exactly in line with the evidence and common eating habits. The average American gets one-third or more of their daily calories from fats, so placing them near the foundation of the pyramid makes sense. Note that it specifically mentions healthy fats and oils, not all types of fat. Good sources of healthy unsaturated fats include olive, canola, soy, corn, sunflower, peanut, and other vegetable oils, trans fat-free margarines, nuts, seeds, avocadoes, and fatty fish such as salmon. These healthy fats not only improve cholesterol levels (when eaten in place of highly processed carbohydrates) but can also protect the heart from sudden and potentially deadly rhythm problems.

Vegetables and Fruits

A diet rich in vegetables and fruits has bountiful benefits. Among them: It can decrease the chances of having a heart attack or stroke; possibly protect against some types of cancers; lower blood pressure; help you avoid the painful intestinal ailment called diverticulitis; guard against cataract and macular degeneration, the major causes of vision loss among people over age 65; and add variety to your diet and wake up your palate.

Nuts, Seeds, Beans, and Tofu

These plant foods are excellent sources of protein, fiber, vitamins, and minerals. Beans include black beans, navy beans, garbanzo, lentils, and other beans that are usually sold dry. Many kinds of nuts contain healthy fats, and packages of some varieties (almonds, walnuts, pecans, peanuts, hazelnuts, and pistachios) can even carry a label saying they're good for your heart.

Fish, Poultry, and Eggs

These foods are also important sources of protein. A wealth of research suggests that eating fish can reduce the risk of heart disease, since fish is rich in heart healthy omega-3 fats. Chicken and turkey are also good sources of protein and can be low in saturated fat. Eggs, which have been demonized because they contain fairly high levels of cholesterol, aren't as bad as they've been cracked up to be. In fact, an egg is a much better breakfast than a doughnut cooked in oil rich in trans fats or a bagel made from refined flour. People with diabetes or heart disease, however, should limit their egg yolk consumption to no more than 3 a week. But egg whites are very high in protein and are a fine substitute for whole eggs in omelets and baking.

Daily (1 to 2 Servings Per Day) or Vitamin D/Calcium Supplements

Building bone and keeping it strong takes calcium, vitamin D, exercise, and a whole lot more. Dairy products have traditionally been Americans' main source of calcium and, through fortification, vitamin D. But most people need at least 1,000 IU of vitamin D per day, far more than the 100 IU supplied by a glass of fortified milk. (See the vitamin section below and in Chapter 9) And there are other healthier ways to get calcium than from milk and cheese, which can contain a lot of saturated fat. Three glasses of whole milk, for example, contains as much saturated fat as 13 strips of cooked bacon. If you enjoy dairy foods, try to stick mainly with no-fat or low-fat products. If you don't like dairy products, taking a vitamin D and calcium supplement offers an easy and inexpensive way to meet your daily vitamin D and calcium needs.

Use Sparingly: Red Meat and Butter

These sit at the top of the Healthy Eating Diet because they contain lots of saturated fat. Eating a lot of red meat may also increase your risk of colon cancer. If you eat red meat every day, switching to fish, chicken, or beans several times a week can improve cholesterol level. So can switching from butter to olive oil. And eating fish has other benefits for the heart.

Use Sparingly: Refined Grains—White Bread, Rice, and Pasta; Potatoes; Sugary Drinks and Sweets; Salt

Why are these all-American staples at the top, rather than the bottom, of the Healthy Eating Pyramid? White bread, white rich, white pasta, other refined grains, potatoes, sugary drinks, and sweets can cause fast and furious increases in blood sugar that can lead to weight gain, diabetes, heart disease, and other chronic disorders. Whole grain carbohydrates cause slower, steadier increases in blood sugar that don't overwhelm the body's ability to handle carbohydrates. The salt shaker is a new addition to the "Use Sparingly" tip of the Healthy Eating Pyramid, one that's based on extensive research linking high-sodium diets to increased risk of heart attack and stroke.

Multivitamin with Extra Vitamin D (For Most People)

A daily multivitamin, multimineral supplement offers a kind of nutritional backup, especially when it includes some extra vitamin D. While a multivitamin can't in any way replace healthy eating, or make up for unhealthy eating, it can fill in the nutritional holes that may sometimes affect even the most careful eaters. You don't need an expensive name-brand or designer vitamin. A standard, store-brand, RDA-level one is fine for most nutrients—except vitamin D. In addition to its bone-health benefit, there's growing evidence that getting some extra vitamin D can help lower the risk of colon and breast cancer. Aim for getting at least 1,000 IU of vitamin D per day: Multiple vitamins are now available with this amount. (Many people, especially those who spend the winter in the Northern U.S. or have darker skin, will need extra vitamin D, often a total of 3,000 to 4,000 IU per day, to bring their blood levels up to an adequate range. (If you are unsure, ask your physician to check your blood level.) Look for a multivitamin that meets the requirements of the USP (U.S. Pharmacopoeia), an organization that sets standards for drugs and supplements.

Optional: Alcohol in Moderation (Not for Everyone)

Scores of studies suggest that having an alcoholic drink a day lowers the risk of heart disease. Moderation is clearly important, since alcohol has risks as well as benefits. For men, a good balance point is one to two drinks a day; in general, however, the risks of drinking even in moderation exceed benefits until middle age. For women, it's at most one drink a day; women should avoid alcohol during pregnancy.

Forget about Numbers and Focus on Quality

You'll notice that the Healthy Eating Pyramid does not give specific advice about the numbers of cups or ounces to have each day of specific foods. That's because it's not meant to be a rigid road map, and the amounts can vary depending on your body size and physical activity. It's a simple, general, flexible guide to how you should eat when you eat.

There's just one basic guideline to remember: A healthy diet includes more foods from the base of the pyramid than from the higher levels of the pyramid. Within this guideline, however, there's plenty of flexibility for different styles of eating and different food choices. A vegetarian can follow the Healthy Eating Pyramid by emphasizing nuts, and other plant sources of protein, and choosing non-dairy sources of calcium and vitamin D: someone who eats animal products can choose fish or chicken for protein, with occasional red meat.

Choosing a variety of fresh, whole foods from all the food groups below the "Use Sparingly" category in the Healthy Eating Pyramid will ensure that you get the nutrients you need. It will also dramatically lower your salt intake, since most of the salt in the U.S. diet lurks in processed food—canned soups, frozen dinners, deli meats, snack chips, and the like.

Perhaps the only foods that are truly off-limits are foods that contain trans fat from partially hydrogenated oils. Luckily, in the U.S. and Canada, trans fats must be listed on nutrition labels. More and more food manufactures, restaurants, and even entire communities are going trans fat-free, making it easier to avoid this health-damaging type of fat.

MyPramid.gov

This interactive website can only be accessed at (http://www.mypyramid.gov), which optimistically means that not more than 42 percent or so of American households with high-speed conductivity can use it—those with slow speed dial-up internet service would find using it very difficult and slow. And of course those without a computer or computer literacy are out of luck all together. This includes many senior citizens.

As for the content of the 2005 Dietary Guidelines for Americans, here's a critique from the Harvard School of Public Health website:

Dietary Guidelines 2005: Two Steps Forward, One Step Back

Released in early January 2005, the Dietary Guidelines for Americans 2005 continues to reflect the tense interplay of science and the powerful food industry. Several of the recommendations in the current version represent important steps in the right direction:

- The current guidelines emphasis the importance of controlling weight, which was not adequately addressed in previous versions. And they continue to stress the importance of physical activity.
- The recommendation on dietary fats makes a clear break from the past, when all fats were considered bad. The guidelines now emphasis that intake of trans fats should be as low as possible and that saturated fat should be limited. There is no longer an artificially low cap on fat intake. The latest advice recommends getting between 20 and 35 percent of daily calories from fats and recognizes the potential health benefits of monounsaturated and polyunsaturated fats.
- Instead of emphasizing "complex carbohydrates," a term used in the past that has little biological meaning, the new guidelines urge Americans to limit sugar intake and stress the benefits of whole grains.

Others remain mired in the past:

- The guidelines suggest that it is fine to consume half of our grains as refined starch. That's a shame, since refined starches, such as white bread and white rice, behave like sugar. They add empty calories, have adverse metabolic effects, and increase the risks of diabetes and heart disease.
- In terms of protein, the guidelines continue to lump together red meat, poultry, fish, and beans (including soy products). They ask us to judge these protein sources by their total fat content, and "make choices that are lean, low-fat, or fat-free." This ignores the evidence that these foods have different types of fats. It also overlooks mounting evidence that replacing red meat with a combination of fish, poultry, beans, and nuts offers numerous health benefits.

♦ The recommendation to drink three glasses of low-fat milk or eat three servings of other dairy products per day to prevent osteoporosis is another step in the wrong direction. Of all the recommendations, this one represents the most radical change from dietary patterns. Three glasses of low-fat milk a day amounts to more than 300 extra calories a day. This is a real issue for the millions of Americans who are trying to

---

MyPyramid Plan

Eat these amounts from each food group daily. This plan is a **2600** calorie food pattern. It is based on average needs for someone like you. (A **70** year old **male**, **5** feet **10** inches tall, of average weight, physically active **more than 60 minutes** a day.) Your calorie needs may be more or less than the average, so check your weight regularly. If you see unwanted weight gain or loss, adjust the amount you are eating.

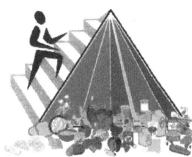

▶ Grains [1]	9 ounces	tips
▶ Vegetables [2]	3.5 cups	tips
▶ Fruits	2 cups	tips
▶ Milk	3 cups	tips
▶ Meat & Beans	6.5 ounces	tips

Click the food groups above to learn more.

[1] **Make Half Your Grains Whole**

Aim for at least 4.5 ounces of whole grains a day

[2] **Vary Your Veggies**

Aim for this much every week:

Dark Green Vegetables = 3 cups weekly
Orange Vegetables = 2 1/2 cups weekly
Dry Beans & Peas = 3 1/2 cups weekly
Starchy Vegetables = 7 cups weekly
Other Vegetables = 8 1/2 cups weekly

Oils & Discretionary Calories

Aim for 8 teaspoons of oils a day

Limit your extras (extra fats & sugars) to 410 Calories

Physical Activity

Physical activity is also important for health. Adults should get at least 30 minutes of moderate level activity most days. Longer or more vigorous activity can provide greater health benefits. Click here to find out if you should talk with a health care provider before starting or increasing physical activity. Click here for more information about physical activity and health.

control their weight. What's more, millions of Americans are lactose intolerant, and even small amounts of milk or dairy products give them stomachaches, gas, or other problems. This recommendation ignores the lack of evidence for a link between consumption of dairy products and prevention of osteoporosis. It also ignores the possible increase in risk of ovarian cancer and prostate cancer associated with dairy products.

The MyPyramid website asks you to enter your age, sex, weight, height, and amount of moderate or vigorous activity. I did that and what follows are the government's recommendations for me.

MyPyramid pegged my daily caloric intake at 2600, which is about what I eat and drink to maintain a healthy weight. All of which proves yet again that the simple rule of energy balance works, and that it matters little where the calories come from, regardless of health ramifications. Otherwise, the faults criticized by the Dr. Willett and the Harvard School of Public Health are there to see. I'm advised to have three cups of milk. I don't. I often have one cup of no-fat milk on cereal or a cup of low-fat yogurt or cottage cheese, never more. I'm advised to have 9 ounces of grains, more than I eat most days—9 ounces is the equivalent of about 7 slices of bread, but I eat more fruits and vegetables than they recommend, which makes up the calorie difference. Then in the footnote they advise me to aim for 4.5 ounces of whole grains, licensing me to eat 4.5 ounces of refined grains, which I know would act on my body as sugar. I now eat refined grains very rarely. Their advice is to eat 6.5 ounces of meat & beans—which ones? We eat a fair amount of fish, poultry, beans, and small portions of lean red meat maybe once or twice a week.

Dr. Willett and his colleagues haven't been mute waiting for the USDA to make corrections. In 2005, *Eat, Drink, and Be Healthy* was republished in a second edition specifically calling attention to the 2005 guidelines faults. In 2008, the Healthy Eating Pyramid was also updated. And I'm confident and hopeful that Dr. Willett will continue to publish. Americans need to know how to enjoy their food and eat defensively. We should be thankful that he and the Harvard School of Public Health are our strong advocates.

Traditional Diets by the Oldways Preservation Trust

As put by Oldways, "These pyramids, taken as a collection, offer substantial refinements of the United States Department of Agriculture's Food Guide Pyramid, refinements that reflect the current state of clinical and epidemiological research world wide and our understanding of what constitutes optimal nutrition status." Essentially, the message is you can eat well and be healthy anywhere in the world; people have until recently been eating traditional foods common to where they live.

It's only in recent years that foods are shipped globally. Throughout history we ate what was available relatively locally. For example, if you lived above the Arctic Circle. Fruits and vegetables were pretty rare, while fish and seal blubber were readily available, so that was the stable food of your diet. Inversely, people in warm climates probably will never eat blubber, but other foods like corn, fruits, and vegetables are readily available. It has to do with the availability of local foods. But these were natural foods and it worked regardless of where you lived. People didn't suffer from the chronic diseases caused by the Western Diet, which is the diet of processed foods and affluence. That's not to say that people weren't undernourished or experienced famine; they did and still do and world famine is a serious problem.

As I wrote earlier my cultural family diet was a blend of Italian/ Mediterranean, German/Jewish, and Pennsylvania Dutch. All challenged in the last twenty years by the promotion of the Western Diet by the food industry—and I gained weight accordingly. The reason why knowing the following traditional food pyramids is important is that you can adopt them and modify them to the Healthy Eating Pyramid very easily and provide variety to your meals. There are differences that you can easily figure out

For instance, the Mediterranean Food Pyramid includes potatoes at the bottom compared to the top of the Healthy Eating Pyramid (in the "use sparingly" category). Also, the Healthy Eating Pyramid emphasizes plant sources of proteins and whole grains. In addition, olive oil and other plant oils are at the bottom of the Healthy Eating Pyramid, whereas olive oil is in the middle of the Mediterranean Pyramid— which I think is mistakenly placed. Our family used a lot of olive oil.

The Healthy Eating Pyramid also recommends a one-a-day vitamin that is missing from the Mediterranean Pyramid.

Probably the biggest difference between the two for me is the type of bread and pastas actually used in Mediterranean cooking. They mostly use semolina flour for bread and pasta, which while delicious, is not a whole grain. We simply substitute whole grains. What follows are the Mediterranean, Asian, Latin American, and vegetarian pyramid; you can make similar substitutions in them all to be in step with the Healthy Eating Pyramid. You can go vegetarian simply by emphasizing nuts, beans, and other plant sources of protein, and choosing non-dairy sources of calcium and vitamin D. Vegans, who eat no animal products at all, have to be particularly careful to get a day's worth of protein— they should also supplement their diets with nutrients that are part of the typical animal protein package, such as vitamin $B_{12,}$ which can be obtained through a standard multivitamin.

Traditional food cookbooks can be a great asset in broadening your diet. You can have fun and enjoy quality foods from many different cultures once you know the fundamentals and stay away from the bad food ingredients.

Eating out, whether Italian, French, Chinese, Japanese, Mexican, Indian, Thai, Greek, American, or the corner deli can be a tricky pleasure. If done infrequently a small indulgence won't kill you. But if you're forced to eat in restaurants frequently, as I was when flying, you have to develop a defensive eating strategy. There are both good and poor choices in all the traditional foods, including ours. Ask the right questions and get what you want and need.

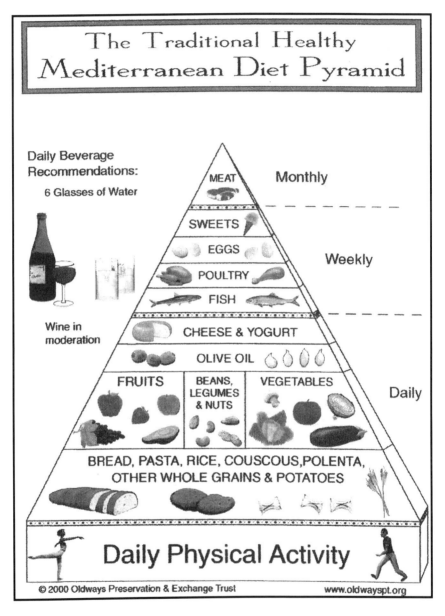

The Traditional Healthy Mediterranean Diet Pyramid

Daily Beverage Recommendations:

6 Glasses of Water

Wine in moderation

MEAT — Monthly

SWEETS
EGGS
POULTRY
FISH — Weekly

CHEESE & YOGURT

OLIVE OIL

FRUITS — BEANS, LEGUMES & NUTS — VEGETABLES — Daily

BREAD, PASTA, RICE, COUSCOUS, POLENTA, OTHER WHOLE GRAINS & POTATOES

Daily Physical Activity

© 2000 Oldways Preservation & Exchange Trust   www.oldwayspt.org

Reproduced with permission from Old Ways Historical Trust

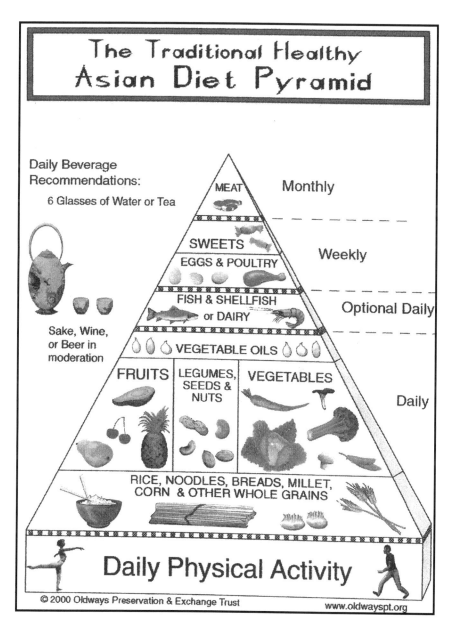

Reproduced with permission from Old Ways Historical Trust

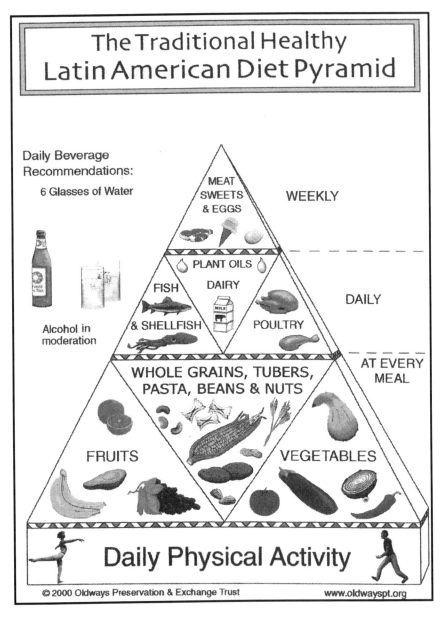

The Traditional Healthy Latin American Diet Pyramid

Daily Beverage Recommendations:

6 Glasses of Water

Alcohol in moderation

MEAT SWEETS & EGGS

WEEKLY

PLANT OILS

FISH & SHELLFISH

DAIRY

POULTRY

DAILY

WHOLE GRAINS, TUBERS, PASTA, BEANS & NUTS

AT EVERY MEAL

FRUITS

VEGETABLES

Daily Physical Activity

© 2000 Oldways Preservation & Exchange Trust   www.oldwayspt.org

Reproduced with permission from Old Ways Historical Trust

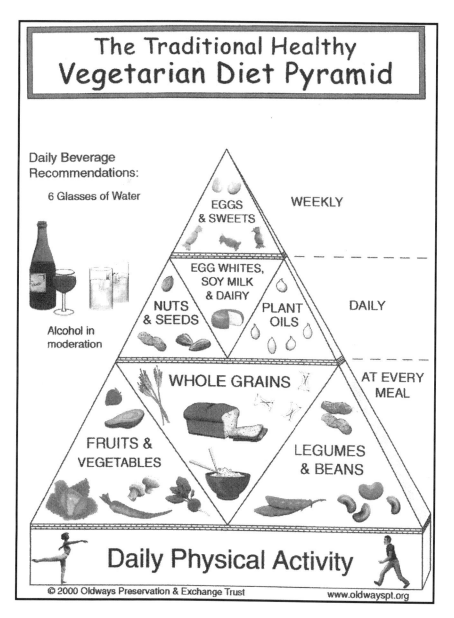

The Traditional Healthy
Vegetarian Diet Pyramid

Daily Beverage
Recommendations:

6 Glasses of Water

Alcohol in
moderation

EGGS
& SWEETS

WEEKLY

EGG WHITES,
SOY MILK
& DAIRY

NUTS
& SEEDS

PLANT
OILS

DAILY

WHOLE GRAINS

AT EVERY
MEAL

FRUITS &
VEGETABLES

LEGUMES
& BEANS

Daily Physical Activity

© 2000 Oldways Preservation & Exchange Trust

www.oldwayspt.org

Reproduced with permission from Old Ways Historical Trust

There are other food pyramids out there as well. Tufts University has a Food Guide Pyramid that is geared to help people 50 years or older—especially those 70 and older. As someone in the latter category, I didn't find it particularly suitable. It seems to be for people considerably less active than I. The Mayo Clinic has one as well. Both are preferable to what the USDA has to offer.

Chapter 13
Keep Your Body Hydrated

As I write this it's an unusually warm day in Northern New Hampshire, about 90 degrees Fahrenheit outdoors and 80 in my office. We don't air condition our home; we need it so rarely that ceiling fans work out fine. Our house sits on a hill and there's usually plenty of airflow—in the winter more than we need. On the plus side, as the price of electricity goes up I can see a wind turbine in our future. But that's another story. At 80 degrees I'm perspiring slightly while doing nothing but sitting at the computer. Perspiration is our body's way of cooling us by the process of evaporation. As usual, I'm slowly sipping a glass of ice water as I write. Sometimes, instead of water, I'll drink hot or cold herbal tea. Shortly, when I stop writing, I'm going to exercise, and after an hour's strenuous row at this room temperature I'll be soaking wet with perspiration. To stay hydrated I'll drink, not sip, more water both during and after my row. I work at staying hydrated; it's one of the things that have helped me lose weight.

Staying hydrated is really about balancing fluid in with fluid out.

Why is staying hydrated important? Remember, over half of our body is liquid, a kind of briny seawater. That fluid is essential to body function. It hydrates our cells, tissues, and organs, carries nutrients, eliminates waste, and enables us to perspire. During my moderately vigorous row, from what the pros say, I'll sweat off about a quart of liquid, which I'll need to replace. Even without exercise on an average day our body loses about half a gallon of liquid a day through sweat, breathing, and urine. During a day's work on a warm day you could easily sweat off a gallon, about 8 pounds, which is the weight of a gallon of water. Whenever you work hard enough to break a good sweat you should take drink breaks, but even with that you'll probably still be slightly dehydrated at the end of the day. Consequently, you'll weigh less, but the majority of that quick weight loss is water, which you'll gain back as you re-hydrate. While exercise and physical activity are essential for good health and weight control, dehydration is not a tool to lose weight. It's a setback. Even mild dehydration is unhealthy; extreme dehydration, like being lost in the desert without water, is life threatening.

If you only drink when you're thirsty the odds are you're slightly dehydrated most of the time, which can make you feel edgy and tired. Experts tell us that chronic dehydration can cause constipation and even kidney stones and bladder cancer. Sure you should drink when thirsty, but by the time you feel thirsty your fluid level can already be too low. You're better off to stay hydrated regardless of thirst, particularly senior citizens, whose sense of thirst is not dependable.

The medical community says we need about a milliliter of fluid for every calorie burned. That works out to about 64 ounces, or 8 glasses (8 ounces) of liquid for a 2,000-calorie-a-day diet. Some of that can come in the foods we eat: melons, fruits, and most vegetables have quite a bit of water. The rest, about 6 glasses, can come from just about anything we drink. Drinking fluids through the day also helps turn off feelings of hunger, making it easier to wait for the next meal, rather than snack.

The next big question is what to drink?

What our body needs is water (H_2O), but that can come packaged with all kinds of stuff, some of it deadly. It's a lot like choosing carbohydrates. The difference between choices can be extreme. For instance, if throughout the day you drink 6 cans of sugared soda you'll add about 900 calories—that's over 6,000 calories a week, guaranteed to pack on almost 2 pounds of fat. In a year it would be 100 pounds!

Just drinking one can (150 calories), if you didn't compensate by eating less, could result in a weight gain of 15 pounds a year. The same amount of water adds no calories at all to your diet. If you need to jazz up the water, add a slice of lemon or a drop or two of fruit juice, or drink herbal tee with no caffeine. Other choices are sparkling water or calorie-free sodas. While the sugar substitutes probably aren't a health hazard for adults, the effect on children is really unknown. For my money putting additional chemicals in your body is unnecessary and foolish. Why do it? I personally don't like sweet drinks.

If you think drinking soda couldn't possibly result in such huge weight gains, think again. Here's one extreme example of what overindulging in junk foods, including sugared sodas can do for you. His name is Manuel Uriba. Mr. Uriba, who now lives in Monterrey, Mexico, said in a recent CNN interview, "that his weight started spiraling out of control when he moved to the United States for a few years in 1988 and indulged in a nonstop diet of junk food and soft drinks." He ultimately grossed out at 1,235 pounds, putting him in the Guinness World Records as the heaviest man in the world. In the past two years, with the help of Dr. Barry Sears, a prescribed Zone diet, and other doctors who are donating their time, he's managed to drop 550 pounds, but is still unable to get out of bed and stand. His goal is to be able to walk down the aisle and marry his fiancée.

Another pointedly deliberate example is the 2004 film, *Super Size Me.* In 2003, Morgan Spurlock filmed a documentary on just how quickly a junk food diet can pack on weight and trash your health; it was nominated for an Academy Award. The stated driving force for Spurlock's investigation was the increasing spread of obesity in the United States, which then Surgeon General Richard Carmona had declared "epidemic," and the corresponding lawsuit brought against McDonald's on behalf of two overweight girls, who, it was alleged, became obese as a result of eating McDonald's food. This was at a time when McDonald's marketing firm, our friends at Porter-Novelli (who did the marketing of MyPyramid), were pushing the "Super Size" theme to get to customers to gorge themselves, and it was working. They did. The lawsuit failed, and subsequently many states have passed legislation prohibiting product liability actions against producers and distributors of "fast food." After *Super Size Me* came out, McDonald's backed away from that advertising campaign. They, of course, still offer every customer the option to Super Size it for a nominal amount of additional money.

Spurlock's film follows a 30-day time period (February 2003), during which he subsists entirely on food and items purchased exclusively at McDonald's. The film documents the drastic effect this lifestyle has on his physical and mental well-being and explores the fast food industry's corporate influence, including how it encourages poor nutrition for its own profit. He dined at McDonald's restaurants three times a day, sampling every item on the chain's menu at least once. He also super sized his meal every time he was asked. He consumed an average of 5,000 calories a day during the experiment.

Before launching the experiment Spurlock was a physically above average 32-year-old, as attested to by three doctors (a cardiologist, a gastroenterologist, and a general practitioner), as well as a nutritionist and a personal trainer. After thirty days, he gained 24.5 pounds, a 13 percent body mass increase, and his Body Mass Index (BMI), rose from 23.2 (within the normal range) to 27 (overweight). He also experienced mood swings, sexual dysfunction, liver damage, and heart palpitations. It took Spurlock fourteen months to lose the weight he gained in a mere thirty days.

Back to drinking choices: about 1/3 of Spurlock's calories came from sugar. In an interview, his nutritionist, Bridget Bennett RD, chided him about his excess intake of sugar from "milkshakes and cokes." All told, they figured he consumed over 30 pounds of sugar from McDonald's.

Sodas and sugared drinks are wasted calories.

While the two cases above are extreme examples, the reality is that people in the United States are getting a large percentage of their carbohydrates from sugared sodas, fruit drinks, and fruit punches. This is not only Super Sizing America, it is creating an epidemic of type II diabetes. This was substantiated by a cohort analysis conducted from 1991 to 1999 among women in the Nurses' Health Study II (Dr. Walter Willett), which found that women who increased their consumption of these drinks gained weight, while those who reduced their consumption lost weight. A follow-up study showed that women who consumed one soda of fruit punch per day increased their risk of type 2 diabetes two-fold. (Journal of the American Medical Association, 2004)

Juice

Eat the fruit or the vegetable—skip the juice. Twelve ounces of pure orange juice contains about 170 calories. It contains the juice and calories of about three oranges, without as much of the fiber. You're better off to eat and orange and, if you're thirsty, drink a glass of water, which is good for you anyway. While you can find pure orange juice most of the other juices are going to come with sugar, usually high-fructose corn syrup; ditto for canned fruit. Vegetable juices like V8 will have salt.

If you really like juice or want to flavor your water start by gradually diluting the juice with water. Eventually you'll find it can be just as satisfying with very little juice and far fewer calories.

Learn to read the labels. Unless fruit juice is first on the list of ingredients, the product is likely to be just sugared water, doctored up to taste like fruit juice.

Coffee and Tea

I like both, but usually only have two cups of coffee in the morning. I never add sugar, and only add skim milk to my coffee when I buy a container for the road to cool it so I don't burn my mouth. I used to ask for an ice cube but found that half the time they'd add a handful and I'd get cold coffee.

Both coffee and tea, with the exception of herbal tea, have caffeine, which is a strong drug that can become addictive. (Tea has less caffeine than coffee.) As an airline captain, I drank a lot of coffee, mostly out of boredom and to stay alert. But this is a two edged sword. It can make you jittery and create an up – down cycle much like sugar. As I got older, I often switched to drinking plain hot water on long transatlantic flights.

The latest science according the Harvard School of Pubic Health is that drinking coffee in moderation is safe and offers some beneficial effects. Coffee tends to lower the risk of developing kidney stones, gallstones, and type 2 diabetes. It also acts as antidepressant and studies show that the suicide rate is 70 percent lower among coffee-drinkers, as opposed to the rate for those who don't drink coffee.

Athletes and Heavy Laborers

While most people in the United States get plenty of salt in prepared foods, strenuous activities on a hot day that causes heavy sweating requires special attention. Our bodies need salt to maintain the proper distribution of fluids inside and outside of cells. If we run low because of heavy sweating, and don't replace the salt, our blood volume goes down, our blood pressure falls; we get weak, and become mentally disorientated. It's a serious condition that if not corrected can kill you.

Most people who do heavy manual labor and athletes are savvy about the need for salt and take some both before and during long events or a hard day's work. Additional glucose helps absorb electrolytes, and prevent hypoglycemia, which can occur after several hours of hard exercise. Marathoners, long distance bike racers, and tennis players will load up on carbohydrates the night before an event for that reason. Some will take sports drinks such as Gatorade that contain sugar, electrolytes, and water to stay hydrated. Another cheaper alternative is to simply take diluted orange juice and a few salty snacks.

Young or old, before you tackle such heavy physical labors you should have a full medical evaluation—it could save your life. We'll focus more on that in Chapter 16.

Chapter 14

Alcohol

The alcoholic beverages that we drink, be it beer, wine, or hard liquors such as gin, whisky, and vodka all contain the alcohol called ethanol, or ethyl alcohol. Ethanol is a toxic substance. Meaning, as soon as you begin to drink alcohol you begin to become intoxicated, at first pleasantly—that's the reason we drink the stuff. Taken in moderation, alcohol is one of life's pleasures: It's relaxing, lowers inhibitions and promotes social exchange, and is now thought to provide important health benefits. However, as you drink more your blood alcohol concentration (BAC) will continue to climb and you'll begin to display intoxicated behavior and eventually get sick, which is far from pleasant or beneficial. If you suck down enough of the stuff, it can kill you by slowing down your heart rate and respiration, and dropping your body temperature. What is "Moderation?" Guidelines are offered in the 2005 Dietary Guidelines for Americans and reiterated later in this chapter under Health Benefits.

Don't drink alcohol when taking certain prescription medications, including sedatives, sleeping pills, and tranquilizers, or taking drugs such as crack cocaine and heroin. Alcohol is a sedative; combined with other sedatives it can put your lights out. You also shouldn't drink while on certain over-the-counter painkillers such as acetaminophen or ibuprofen because it can be extremely harmful to your liver and stomach.

Alcoholics, or those with a family history of alcoholism, are advised not to drink at all, because alcohol can be addictive. For these, one drink is too many and polishing off a bottle is not enough. Whether a diagnosed alcoholic or not, heavy drinking can wreck your life, destroy your liver, kidneys and heart, and put you in an early grave. According to national surveys by the Centers for Disease Control and Prevention (CDC), over half of the adult population of the U.S. drinks alcohol. Approximately 5 percent of this population drinks heavily, while 15 percent of the population binge drinks. (Heavy drinking is typically defined as drinking more than two drinks a day on average for men, and one drink a day for women. Binge drinking is consuming more than five drinks on a single occasion for men, and four drinks for women.) The CDC further reports that from 2001-2005 there were approximately 79,000 deaths annually attributed to excessive alcohol use. Driving while intoxicated (BAC greater than 0.08) was responsible for 13,990 deaths in 2006, as reported by the U.S. Department of Transportation

Fermentation and Distillation

Despite the dark sides of alcohol, of which there are many, people have been drinking and fermenting alcohol (ethanol) for a long, long time. In Egypt, the discovery of late Stone Age beer jugs has established the fact that fermented beverages existed at least as early as the Neolithic period (10,000 BC), and it has been suggested that beer may have preceded bread as a staple. Wine clearly appeared as a finished product in Egyptian pictographs around 4,000 BC. Evidence of the use of alcoholic beverages also comes from China, India, Babylon, Greece, and Pre-Columbian America.

Fermentation occurs naturally in nature. For instance, many berries break open in the late fall when they are overripe and full of sugar. Natural yeast organisms lodge on the surface of these berries, which then become fermented and alcoholic. Perhaps that's why bears go for a long winter's sleep, and why birds sometimes fly so erratically—who knows?

Fermentation is the conversion of sugar to alcohol, using yeast under anaerobic (in the absence of oxygen) conditions—it's the chemical conversion of carbohydrates into alcohol, acids, and carbon dioxide. The process is used to produce wine, beer, and cider, and to begin the process of producing alcoholic spirits. It is also used to create lactic acid to preserve sour foods such as pickled cucumbers, kimchi (a Korean dish) and yogurt. Fermentation also produces carbon dioxide to leaven bread.

And, believe it or not, the human body normally produces small amounts of endogenous ethanol from sugars in the intestines that are fermented by intestinal flora (microorganisms that inhabit our digestive systems). In some rare cases, Candidiasis (a yeast infection) in the intestines, or short bowel syndrome (SBS), can result in what's called "auto-brewery syndrome," a term used to describe patients who show signs of alcohol intoxication because of abnormal yeast growth after ingesting carbohydrate-rich meals. At this point, scientists really aren't sure of the role endogenous ethanol plays in the body's overall metabolism, but some think it may be significant.

Humans, like other critters, also produce methane gas, along with sulfa and other gases, as the result of the fermentation in the digestive system, which is excreted as flatulence. Worldwide more than 1.3 billion cows belching and farting are contributing enough methane (a potent greenhouse gas) to be a major factor in global warming. Cows, which are ruminates, eat a tremendous amount of carbohydrates. There are 100 million cows in the United States alone, and, as China and other countries develop a taste for red meat, the bovine population can be expected to increase, exacerbating the problem. Methane gas is chemically a fossil fuel, so along with fermenting ethanol in our bodies it can be said that we humans are fossil fuels producers (ethanol and methane gas) as well as consumers, all involved in metabolism and the burning of fuel for energy. It's an extremely complicated and elegant cycle.

Distillation is the process used to separate mixtures that contain at least one liquid. It works because each substance in the mixture has its own unique boiling point. With alcoholic beverages, distillation is used to increase the percentage of ethanol within an already fermented mixture (distillation itself does not make alcohol). Even repeated fermentation by adding yeast cannot raise the percentage of alcohol to more than 17 percent because yeasts for human consumption cannot grow in a higher mixture. Distillation can produce liquors that range from 40-95 percent ethyl alcohol. The amount of alcohol in any one beverage varies. There are differences in the amount of alcohol between beer, wine, champagne, and distilled spirits (those that contain more than 30 percent alcohol). The amount of alcohol is given as a percentage and also in "proof." The proof of an alcoholic beverage is equal to twice the percentage of ethyl alcohol contained—therefore 100 proof ethanol is 50 percent alcohol and 50 proof is 25 percent, etc. Following is the alcoholic content of various beverages:

Beverage	Percentage Alcohol	Proof
Beer	4 – 6	8 – 12
Wine	7 – 15	14 – 30
Champagne	4 – 14	16 – 28
Distilled Spirits	40 – 95	80 – 190

Most distilled spirits on the market are 80 proof; some top shelve brands are 90+ proof, and a very few are 100 proof. To buy higher proof natural spirits usually requires a special permit from the state liquor commission. Proofs in excess of 110 are dangerous to drink casually, if not watered down. Taken straight they can burn your month, esophagus, and wreck your stomach.

Universally a "drink" is considered to be 12 ounces of beer, or 5 ounces of wine, or 1.5 ounces of distilled spirits. While the number of alcohol calories in each beverage is the same, about 97 calories, the total number of calories is quite different: gin, rum, vodka, and whiskey is mostly water diluted pure alcohol and remains 97 calories; wine contains about 114 calories, and regular beer about 153 calories. The difference in calories is the non-fermented contents, the grapes, the malts, and so forth, which are carbohydrates. That's an important distinction; we'll learn why shortly. It somewhat explains the proverbial beer belly.

The distillation of alcohol can be traced back to China, Central Asia and the Middle East. Some archaeological evidence suggests that the practice of distillation in China may date back to 5,000 BC. Muslim chemists were the first to produce fully purified alcohol in the 8th and 9th centuries. The terms "alembic" and "alcohol", and possibly the metaphors "spirit" and *aqua vita* ("life-water") for the distilled product can be traced back to Arabic alchemy. Early use of distilled alcohol was for medicine, but by the mid-12th century it had spread to Europe and the use of distilled alcoholic beverages was well under way.

The Beneficial Effects of Alcohol

The reason alcohol has been with us so long is because it's pleasurable to drink, and throughout most of history, despite the known dangers, it has been considered a gift from God. It was also often safer to drink wine and beer than water. It's still safer in many places. The availability of pure water is yet another world crisis that looms. Wine or beer is preferable to questionably bad water because the process of fermentation kills or weakens bacteria. Distilled alcohol kills bacteria and, if properly sealed, can be stored for years. In fact, many wines and spirits improve with age. For thousands of years people intuitively knew that a moderate amount of alcohol was good for you. In recent years modern science has come to the same conclusion for some, but not all people.

Alcohol's complex role in human health and nutrition is very unique. Unlike the macronutrients fats, carbohydrates and protein, which have nutrients and calories, alcohol has only calories. No nutrients. Some nutritionists list alcohol together with the micronutrients because more than half of the adults in the U.S. get 10 percent or more of their daily calories from it. Although not a nutrient, alcohol is an energy source capable of providing calories for all essential biological activities, including replication, functions and maintenance of individual cells, energy for physical work, and thermogenesis (the process by which the body produces heat). But there are several outstanding differences between alcohol and the macronutrients:[5]

+ A gram of pure alcohol has 7 calories of energy, almost twice that of carbohydrates and protein, which have 4 calories of energy. Fats have 9 calories of energy. Although high in energy, alcohol has no nutrients—it's why alcoholics and heavy drinkers are often undernourished, thin, and suffer from vitamin deficiencies.

+ Unlike excess fat calories, carbohydrate calories, and protein calories, the body has no ability to store alcohol calories. Carbohydrates and protein are turned into glucose. Some of the glucose goes into the bloodstream and is used for energy, some is stored as glycogen in muscles and the liver, and what's left over gets converted to fat and stored in fat cells to be burned when your body doesn't have enough food or glycogen. Alcohol is unique; its calories are either used for energy or excreted as CO_2 and water. But don't be misled. If you drink and eat heavy, unhealthy meals, your body will burn what alcohol it can and still store the food calories as body fat—the total number of calories from any source count.

+ Our body's fuel consumption is prioritized largely by the regulation of entry of the energy source into the cells. For sugars (carbs), fatty acids (fats), and amino acids (protein), this transport across the plasma membrane is mediated by proteins made by the body. In contrast, alcohol freely diffuses across plasma membranes, not requiring protein-mediated transport. The liver, by use of enzymes, offers alcohol about a ten-step short cut in its conversion to a molecule called adenosine triphosphate (ATP), which is the singular source of energy for all cells. As a result, alcohol has a unique role and hierarchal position in human nutrition.

+ While alcohol is a concentrated source of calories, it is no longer in its pre-fermented chemical state as a carbohydrate and does not get converted into sugar. It therefore does not raise blood sugar levels and does not require insulin in the blood stream to deal with it. Ethanol has a glycemic index of zero. If the alcohol is packaged with sugared drinks, like coke or ginger ale, it's of course a different story; sugared drinks contain lots of carbohydrates.

If you take insulin or certain medications to control diabetes, drinking alcohol can put you at risk for low blood sugar, a condition called hypoglycemia. (Your body, particularly your brain, still needs glucose to function.) This is especially true if you drink on an empty stomach or don't have adequate carbohydrates because alcohol also reduces your body's ability to mobilize glucose from stored body fat.

The short of it is that alcohol plays a part in human metabolism, some of which is known, and much of which, it seems, has yet to be learned. It's been determined by statistical analysis that the health benefits from alcohol can be attributed to the alcohol itself, not to red wine packaging, which was the reason some credited the French diet as healthy. Although the French and other Mediterranean meals can be high in fat, they're almost always accompanied by red wine—yet the rate of heart disease in France and in some other Mediterranean countries is far lower than in the United States.

Since alcohol has virtually no nutritional value, it stands to reason that the health benefits of alcohol have to be related to its sedative and relaxing property. Modern life is hugely stressful and relieving that stress is beneficial. Moderate use of alcohol may even relieve the stress associated with trying to change dietary habits and lose weight. Exercise is a great way to relieve stress as well.

The medical community's recommendations concerning the health benefits of moderate alcohol use are based on the statistical outcomes of large group studies, including Dr. Willett's 40,000-man study. The underlying physiological reasons why seem to be speculative at best. (*Eat, Drink, and Be healthy*)

In January 1997, the National Institute on Alcohol Abuse and Alcoholism of the National Institute of Health published the most concise, authoritative explanation of alcohol metabolism I have come across. Parts of the *Alcohol Alert* follow:

Alcohol Metabolism

Metabolism is the body's process of converting ingested substances to other compounds. Metabolism results in some substances becoming more, and some less, toxic than those originally ingested. Metabolism involves a number of processes, one of which is referred to as oxidation. Through oxidation, alcohol is detoxified and removed from the blood, preventing the alcohol from accumulating and destroying cells and organs. A minute amount of alcohol escapes metabolism and is excreted unchanged in the breath and in urine. As this *Alcohol Alert* explains, by understanding alcohol metabolism, we can learn how the body can dispose of alcohol and discern some of the factors that influence this process. Studying alcohol metabolism also can help us to understand how this process influences the metabolism of food, hormones, and medications.

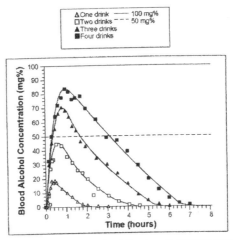

Blood alcohol concentration (BAC) after the rapid consumption of different amounts of alcohol by eight adult fasting male subjects.* (Adapted from Wilkinson et al., *Journal of Pharmacokinetics and Biopharmaceutics* 5(3):207-224, 1977.)

100 mg% is the legal level of intoxication in most States. 50 mg% is the level at which deterioration of driving skills begins. *(JAMA* 255:522-527, 1986.)

If the same number of drinks are consumed over a longer period of time, BAC's will be lower.

The Metabolic Process

When alcohol is consumed, it passes from the stomach and intestines into the blood, a process referred to as absorption. Alcohol is then metabolized by enzymes, which are body chemicals that break down other chemicals. In the liver, an enzyme called alcohol dehydrogenase (ADH) mediates the conversion alcohol to acetaldehyde. Acetaldehyde is rapidly converted to acetate by other enzymes and is eventually metabolized to carbon dioxide and water. Alcohol also is metabolized in the liver by the enzyme cytochrome P450011E1 (CYP2E1), which may be increased after chronic drinking. Most of the alcohol consumed is metabolized in the liver, but the small quantity that remains unmetabolized permits alcohol concentrations to be measured in breath and urine.

The liver can metabolize only a certain amount of alcohol per hour, regardless of the amount that has been consumed. The rate of alcohol metabolism depends, in part, on the amount of metabolizing enzymes in the liver, which varies among individuals and appears to have genetic determinants. [For example, Asians apparently don't produce much ADH and have a very low tolerance of alcohol.] In general, after the consumption of one standard drink, the amount of alcohol in the drinker's blood (blood alcohol concentration, or BAC) peaks within 30 to 45 minutes. (A standard drink is defined as 12 ounces of beer, 5 ounce of wine, or 1.5 ounces of 80-proof distilled spirits, all of which contain the same amount of alcohol.) The BAC curve, shown on the previous page, provides an estimate of the time needed to absorb and metabolize different amounts of alcohol. Alcohol is metabolized more slowly than it is absorbed. Since the metabolism of alcohol is slow, consumption needs to be controlled to prevent accumulation in the body and intoxication.

The medical community now seems to agree, however, that moderate drinking for most adults may be beneficial. Excluded are pregnant women, those with a history of hemorrhagic stroke, liver disease, pancreatic disease, evidence of precancerous changes in the esophagus, larynx, pharynx or mouth, and those with a family history of alcoholism.

The experts also caution that the benefits of drinking alcohol are quickly reversed if you drink heavily. There's universal agreement that heavy drinking and binge drinking are bad for you. Also, having six drinks on a Saturday night and abstaining during the week has no health benefit at all. All you get to do is lose a weekend.

As said earlier, certain prescription and over-the-counter drugs can interact with alcohol badly. The answer is to discuss the pros and cons for you with your doctor—more on why in Chapter 16. The following list of benefits can be found at MayoClinic.com:

Health Benefits

Moderate alcohol consumption may provide some health benefits. It may:

- Reduce your risk of developing heart disease, peripheral vascular disease and intermittent claudication.
- Reduce your risk of dying of a heart attack.
- Possibly reduce your risk of strokes, particularly ischemic strokes.
- Lower your risk of gallstones.
- Possibly reduce your risk of diabetes.

As a general guideline for healthy adults with no family history of alcoholism, moderation means up to two drinks a day for men and one for women and older people. (Source: 2005, Dietary Guidelines for Americans)

Women appear to metabolize alcohol slower, and are, on average, smaller, thus having less blood to dilute the alcohol.

My Personal View

To me, moderate drinking, like sex, is one of life's great pleasures. And like sex, without moderation and good judgment, drinking can wreck your life and kill you. It's not only a matter of self-discipline, it's a matter of education. My parents set an example for me. My father always had decanted red wine on the table for dinner, but I never saw him drunk. On holidays, as a child I'd get a small amount of wine in a large glass of cream soda. Consequently alcohol was never a taboo and the children in our extended family learned to drink responsibly and in moderation. Drunkenness was not socially acceptable.

The same example was set about sex. Simply put, my father was a gentleman and treated mother with open love and respect. There were no lectures about abstinence of either sex or alcohol; it would have been totally irrelevant. I was expected to both grow up and enjoy life, and to be a responsible human being. Teaching our children abstinence instead of birth control and human sexuality doesn't work any better than preaching the evils of alcohol. As a nation we have to give our children confident skills to know how to live, eat, and drink. They're going to do it all anyway, whether we like it or not.

Jerry's Tips

- Always combine drinking with great meals. With food in your stomach, you'll absorb the alcohol slower and naturally drink less.
- Stay away from appetizers, particularly junk bar foods such as pretzels and potato chips, when you drink. You can easily get more calories from these than from a couple of drinks, and ruin your dinner to boot. If you need something to nosh on eat a few nuts or celery as I do.
- Don't drink after dinner. An occasional after dinner cordial with guests is fine, but it should be infrequent or you'll kick up your daily calorie intake needlessly. If you want something sweet after dinner, have a piece of fruit.
- Dilute hard liquor (gin, whisky, vodka) with water and/or ice. Drinking 80 proof spirits "neat" (straight) frequently is dangerous—it's an irritant that can cause cancer. Aside from my Sunday Bloody Mary, I dilute my gin with ice water—instructions later. If you need other mixers make them no-cal.

- Personally, I enjoy wine with a meal, but rarely drink beer because of the additional calories.
- Use reasonably sized glasses. Most of us don't measure when we pour at home. If you use a fish bowl, and think you're only having one or two, you're not being moderate, you're just kidding yourself.
- At parties learn to recognize the different stages of intoxication. If someone is slurring words, or stumbling, they've had too much to drink to drive safely. Know and respect the BAC time chart given in the *Alcohol Alert*.
- If drinking is interfering with your work or relationships you have a problem. Cut back, and get help if you can't. If you need help, start with your doctor. He or she can point you in the right direction.

Jerry's Martini on the Rocks

My gin of choice is Tanqueray, a London Dry Gin that's 94.6 proof.

Start by filling an 8-ounce tumbler with ice cubes.

Then put a few cubes in a cocktail shaker and add about a half-ounce of extra dry white vermouth; I use Martini and Rossi.

Pour about 2 ounces of gin over the rocks in the tumbler—this will bring the fluid level up to about two-thirds because the glass is filled with ice.

Twirl the vermouth in the shaker and empty it down the drain—the vermouth coating the shaker is plenty for a dry martini.

Dump the contents of the tumbler into the shaker and using another 12-ounce glass placed into the shaker, shake well. The idea is to make the drink super cold and melt some of the ice.

Pour the whole works back into the tumbler.

You can use the traditional olive or a lemon twist but I prefer a big stalk of cold celery on the side to munch on; it puts food in your stomach that has few calories and tons of water.

If you sip the drink until the glass is empty and the cubes are gone you'll have diluted the gin with over 5 ounces of water—a far better choice than drinking the martini straight up in a cocktail glass.

If you want to get wild and crazy add some raspberries—it tastes and looks great. I call that version a "Rasputin."

To Life!

Chapter 15

Physical Activity and Exercise

The Flip Side of the Equation

We know the equation, if calories in equal calories out (burned) we maintain a weight. If we tip that balance either way we'll either gain or lose weight. We've learned that, next to not smoking, weight control is the single most important factor in staying healthy. And that physical activity is an essential part of controlling your weight. We spent a lot of time learning about food; now let's focus on the other side of the equation—the health benefits of physical activity and exercise, which go far beyond just burning off careless calories. Then we'll move on to ways to be more physically active and the need to exercise.

Throughout human history obesity and lack of physical activity were only a problem for the nobility. The rest of us had to do hard physical labor just to get the essentials of life. Very few of us do the kind of work today that increases your heart rate, gets you breathing hard, and works up a sweat. I certainly didn't. Although I piloted aircraft that weighed hundreds of thousands of pounds, the only weight I ever physically lifted at work was my overnight bag and flight kit. The rest of the time I sat on my butt. Most people don't do any more physical work than I did professionally, or for that mater as I do now sitting at the computer. For the most part, in industrial nations, machines have replaced hard, physical labor.

By the 1990s, just about everybody in the medical community recognized that Americans were physically falling apart. Obesity and lack of physical activity was epidemic. With an eye to the problem, in 1994, then Secretary of Health and Human Services Donna E. Shalala, commissioned the first Surgeon General's report on physical activity and health. The report was prepared with the combined efforts of the Department of Health and Human Services, Centers for Disease Control and Prevention, National Center for Chronic Disease Prevention and Health Promotion, and The President's Council on Physical Fitness and Sports.

The Surgeon General's report was released with a lot of press coverage on the eve of the Summer Centennial Olympic Games in Atlanta Georgia in 1996. The findings on the levels of physical activity for Americans were shocking. The report's recommendations constituted a landmark change in public policy. Up until this report, the Dietary Guidelines for Americans were silent on the benefits of exercise. That wouldn't change until 2005. The Executive Summary of the report can be found at: http://www.cdc.gov/nccdphp/sgr/summary.htm

Major Conclusions of the Report

1. People of all ages, both male and female, benefit from regular physical activity.

2. Significant health benefits can be obtained by including a moderate amount of physical activity (e.g., 30 minutes of brisk walking or raking leaves, 15 minutes of running, or minutes of playing volleyball) on most, if not all, days of the week. Through a modest increase in daily activity, most Americans can improve their health and quality of life.

3. Additional health benefits can be gained through greater amounts of physical activity. People who can maintain a regular regimen of activity that is of longer duration or more vigorous intensity are likely to derive greater benefits.

4. *Physical activity reduces the risk of premature mortality in general, and of coronary heart disease, hypertension, colon cancer, and diabetes mellitus in particular. Physical activity also improves mental health and is important for the health of muscles, bones, and joints.* [Emphasis is mine.]

5. More than 60 percent of American adults are not regularly physically active. In fact, 25 percent of adults are not active at all.

6. Nearly half of American youths 12-21 years of age are not vigorously active on a regular basis. Moreover, physical activity declines dramatically during adolescence.

7. Daily enrollment in physical education classes has declined among high school students from 42 percent in 1991 to 25 percent in 1995.

8. Research on understanding and promoting physical activity is at an early stage, but some interventions to promote physical activity through schools, worksites, and health care settings have been evaluated and found to be successful.

Unfortunately, the optimism expressed in the report's conclusions hasn't panned out. As this is written, twelve years after the report was published, the numbers haven't improved. They've gotten worse. Obesity and lack of physical activity remain at record levels in the United States. Globally, our exported Western diet and reduced physical activity—life styles joined at the hip—has created over 3 billion overweight adults, with at least 300 million of them obese.[6] The resulting epidemic of chronic diseases in the United States is responsible for one-third of the years of potential life lost before age 65. Without a change in the way we eat and exercise, this generation of Americans may be the first to have a shorter life expectancy than their parents. And perhaps worse than an early death, the quality of life for those years that we live continues to deteriorate as chronic disease strikes more and more of us—in 2000 about 133 million Americans, 45 percent, had at least one chronic disease.

When we consider that 75 percent of the cost of healthcare in the United States is attributed to the treatment of chronic diseases, which can be mitigated or avoided by not smoking, weight control, and exercise, the financial burden of poor personal health choices is staggering. In 2007, health care spending in the United States reached $2.3 trillion, and is expected to reach $3 trillion in 2011, and projected to reach $4.2 trillion by 2016. For the individual, medical bills and health insurance have become a major cost of living and are one of the leading causes of bankruptcy. Our healthcare system is broken, the costs are unsustainable, and the outcomes pathetically poor for the money spent. If you don't want to become a sad statistic, you have to get moving and make exercise an enjoyable part of every day. I sure do.

If you're a senior citizen as I am, one of our greatest concerns as we grow older isn't immortality—nobody lives forever—it's to be able to live independently, and to be able to continue doing the things we enjoy. I'm reminded of a beautiful advertisement that British actress Lynn Redgrave made for Bristol-Myers Squibb concerning breast cancer; Ms. Redgrave is a breast cancer survivor. Here's the way she put it:

I want to die from eating too much chocolate.
I want to die from exhaustion from dancing the tango.
I want to die from laughing too hard on my 87th birthday.
I refuse to die from breast cancer.

I refuse to die from being overweight. So should you. If you're overweight and need the incentive to get started on an exercise program, I recommend visiting a nursing home. Nursing homes provide skilled nursing care for those who are incapable of living independently, and for those who need long term care to recover from illness or injuries. For the past three months I've been visiting a dear friend who's recovering from a leg amputation and several associated maladies in a Veterans Administration nursing home. He's a vet.

The first thing that you'll notice is that the vast majority of patients suffers from obesity and/or has very little mobility. Many will be in wheel chairs. Although the staff won't discuss individual cases, they'll candidly tell you that almost all the residents are being treated for multiple chronic diseases—treatments that for the most part will not restore their ability to live independently. I suggest you look back into your past and then fast-forward into your future as Ebenezer Scrooge did in *A Christmas Carol*. Think of your ability to function as a kid or in college, and then of what your life will be like if you continue to gain weight and be inactive. The question is, do you want to spend your golden years unable to care for yourself living in an institution. It's your choice. Scrooge changed his ways and got a second chance. So can you. I'm here to tell you that you'll love it. Before long there'll be no more huffing and puffing going up a flight of stairs (or having sex, which you may have given up), and many of those aches, pains, and difficulties you have in getting around will fade. It won't happen overnight, but it will happen.

My buddy at the VA hospital is doing well. Obesity is not his problem. It will take time, but he'll eventually get out of the joint. He's working at it.

The Relationship Between Exercise, Fat, and Muscles

We know that exercise burns calories that would otherwise be stored as fat. And that exercise builds muscles. Here's the rest of the story on why exercise is an essential part of weight control.

Remember the discussion on basal metabolic rate (BMR)? It refers to the calories your body burns even while at rest, which accounts for two-thirds to three quarters of the calories burned each day. Of course, muscles burn more calories when you exercise, but they also burn calories when you're doing nothing, far more calories than fat cells, which burn very few calories no matter what you're doing. So the ratio of muscle or lean body mass to body fat is an extremely important factor in maintaining a healthy weight. The only way you can build those muscles is by regular physical activity and/or exercise. Although the terms have been used interchangeably, there is a difference that we'll discuss shortly.

It logically follows that a sedentary lifestyle limits the number of calories that can be consumed without gaining weight. The more a person exercises, the higher his or her energy requirement, and the easier it is to plan daily meals that don't exceed your caloric needs.

Inversely, if you're sedentary, your muscles shrink, as do your caloric needs, and unless you eat less, which most people don't manage to do, those excess calories get stored as fat. As your body composition ratio tips toward more fat and less lean body mass (muscle), your metabolism (BMR) slows down, and you begin a vicious cycle that makes it easier to gain weight and harder to lose it. Some say that's just a natural part of growing older. Baloney. It's a natural part of growing older if you don't keep moving and exercising.

Keep Track of Body Fat

Here's why your regular bathroom scale doesn't tell you the complete story. If you're a couch potato, a weight gain of 15 pounds over a couple of years might actually be a gain of 25 pounds of fat and a loss of 10 pounds of muscle. That's the reason why I recommended earlier in Chapter 1 investing in a Body Composition Analyzer; it not only gives you an accurate weight, it also measures your percentage of body fat. If you're serious about attaining a healthy weight, you need to know both.

Getting Started

Following up on the Surgeon General's report on physical fitness in 1996, the Dietary Guidelines for Americans 2005 made specific recommendations concerning physical activity. Physical activity is defined as any bodily movement produced by skeletal muscles resulting in energy expenditure. The complete text can be found at: http://www.health.gov/DietaryGuidelines/dga2005/document/html/chapter4.htm

Key Recommendations

- Engage in regular physical activity and reduce sedentary activities to promote health, psychological well-being, and a healthy body weight.
  - o To reduce the risk of chronic disease in adulthood: Engage in at least 30 minutes of moderate-intensity physical activity, above usual activity, at work or home on most days of the week.
  - o For most people, greater health benefits can be obtained by engaging in physical activity of more vigorous intensity or longer duration.
  - o To help manage body weight and prevent gradual, unhealthy body weight gain in adulthood: Engage in approximately 60 minutes of moderate-to vigorous-intensity activity on most days of the week while not exceeding caloric intake.
  - o To sustain weight loss in adulthood: Participate in at least 60 to 90 minutes of daily moderate-intensity physical activity while not exceeding caloric intake requirements. *Some people may need to consult with a healthcare provider before participating in this level of activity.* [Emphasis is mine.]
- Achieve physical fitness by including cardiovascular conditioning, stretching exercises for flexibility, and resistance exercises or calisthenics for muscle strength and endurance.

Key Recommendations for Specific Population Groups

- *Children and adolescents.* Engage in at least 60 minutes of physical activity on most, preferably all, days of the week.
- *Pregnant women.* In the absence of medical or obstetric complications, incorporate 30 minutes or more of moderate-intensity physical activity on most, if not all, days of the week. Avoid activities with a high risk of falling or abdominal trauma.
- *Breastfeeding women.* Be aware that neither acute nor regular exercise adversely affects the mother's ability to successfully breastfeed.

• *Older adults. Participate in regular physical activity to reduce functional declines associated with aging and to achieve the other benefits of physical activity identified for all adults.* [Emphasis is mine.]

I've emphasized the recommendation to consult a healthcare provider because I personally feel that everyone should have routine annual physicals and that everyone should consult their physician before starting any kind of moderate to vigorous exercise program, particularly those with known medical problems. I've also emphasized the bullet on the additional benefits for older adults who exercise—being one; I'm walking proof that it works.

Not being sedentary enables you to glean the benefits of physical activity in your everyday routines. People still need regular exercise above what you do at work or home, but simply not sitting on your duff when you can move is a free-bee. One of the biggies is not to spend hours sitting in front of a TV set. A lot of the TV I watch is while exercising. Try it. It's great. I have a TV in my gym area, but you can do a lot of simple resistance exercises, like stomach crunches, push ups, and arm curls with small weights right in your living room and still enjoy a show. It's a heck of a lot better than sitting and snacking on junk food.

For children, too much TV has been a killer. The Behavioral Risk Factor Surveillances System (BRFSS) reported that in 2002, 25 percent of adult Americans did not participate in any leisure time physical activities in the past month, and in 2003, 38 percent of students in grades 9 to 12 viewed television 3 or more hours per day. And, if you've noticed, the junk-food peddlers know the kids are watching. Look at the ads they run, particularly around meal times.

These days sedentary time at the computer is also problematic. Kids are playing computer games or blogging when they should be outside playing. While I don't play video games or blog, I do quite a bit of work at the computer, including many disciplined hours writing. What saves me is that I make a point of frequently getting up and moving around.

When my mind starts turning to mashed potatoes, I know it's time work out. My gym area is right next to my office.

There are many simple things you can work into your daily routine to increase physical activity. I have a friend and neighbor who's a very senior executive at large local business that employs hundreds of workers. Certainly he rates a reserved parking space near the door. But he doesn't use one. Instead he parks the farthest away from the entrance he can get, although he's usually among the first to be at work in the morning. He prefers the walk, and, incidentally, usually hits the health club for a workout before he gets to work. He's in his sixties and in great shape. Juxtaposed, we live in a relatively small town with a main street that only stretches less than a mile. Yet people routinely will stop and park several times, rather than once and enjoying the walk. On the other hand, I know others who eat a small lunch and briskly walk the rest of their lunch hour. Guess which ones look the fittest.

There are plenty of things you can do to keep moving: skip the elevator, take the stairs; mow the grass, rake the leaves; walk the dog; play with your children or grandchildren; if you're a desk jockey, get up and pace or dance around. It's good for your circulation. The list is almost endless.

Exercise and physical activity: What's the difference?

As said earlier, the terms physical activity and exercise are often used interchangeably, but there are important differences. As defined in the Dietary Guidelines for Americans, physical activity is "...any bodily movement produced by skeletal muscles resulting in energy expenditure." This includes both aerobic and anaerobic activities (more later). These are the type of physical activity people do for recreation (sports), transportation (walking or riding a bike), or work, including household chores.

Exercise is actually a subcategory of physical activity. It's a structured program of physical activity for attaining fitness for health reasons and/or athletic performance. All professional athletes exercise—just playing the sport, whichever it be, is not sufficient physical training to functionally excel in most sports. I was a lower level professional ski instructor. If I didn't exercise away from the mountain, I couldn't do the job. Bode Miller, who's been the resident ski racing champ at Bretton Woods, the ski mountain I taught at, is noted for his exercise regimen—he was brought up and lives in the hereby town of Eastern. Tiger Woods is another example; his golfing excellence is a combination of talent, skills, and physical fitness maintained by exercise away from the golf course.

Even for those physically active, structured exercise can increase your total energy expenditure, help you lose weight, and improve your overall conditioning and health.

What is physical fitness?

In setting your goals and measuring your progress, you really need to known how fit you actually are. Otherwise you'll backslide. One measure is the amount of oxygen your body can use. Another is functional fitness, which requires a healthy heart, lungs, muscles, and bones. For most of us, who are not professional athletes, this is what counts—to be able to do things. Look around in any public place and you'll see those who are barely functional. That's not where you want to be.

Exercise

Somewhere along the line we've all been required to "exercise." In grammar school, in my memory, the kids were just let out in the school playground twice a day for fifteen minutes to run around and play—hardly structured exercise, but it was a way for the kids to move and burn off energy. In high school, it used to be that physical training was a required course in every semester. It is no longer. Now, in most high school curriculums, only one semester is required in the entire four years. There's so much pressure on "no child left behind," and the rest of what modern society seems to expect academically, that exercise and health take a back seat. It's an incredibly stupid value judgment.

If you ever served in the armed forces, you learned about exercise the hard way through basic training. Today basic training in the United States Army incorporates a vigorous regimen of physical training. If you're interested, you can find the Army's Physical Training Guide at:

http://assets.goarmy.com/downloads/pocket_pt_guide.pdf It's a program meant for young recruits, certainly not senior citizens or long time couch potatoes.

For those who have never been involved in a structured exercise program of any kind I recommend joining a health club. They all have qualified fitness coaches who can help you get started. They're not that expensive to hire for a few sessions, and it's a great way to learn how to exercise properly. Of course just briskly walking, jogging, or bike riding is great exercise, but for you to get the most benefit from the time spent, it will take some training or a great deal of personal research to accomplish.

Moderate Intensity

Years back, when I started exercising as an adult in the 1960s, the word was "no pain, no gain," and high-intensity exercise was emphasized for cardiovascular fitness. We've since learned that's not true. First, moderate-intensity exercise offers substantial health benefits. Second, most people, including senior citizens, simply aren't willing to hit it that hard. Sure, if you're inclined to push a bit, go for it. It can be fun. I do sometimes, but not all the time, and never to my absolute limit. It's much more important that we exercise on a regular daily basis. It has to be a pleasurable part of your life. You gain strength and stamina each day you exercise—you begin to lose it when you stop. This is particularly so with aerobic exercise or endurance exercise. Muscle strength from anaerobic or resistance training fades at a slower rate.

Frequency and Duration

I think the advice from the Dietary Guidelines for Americans is right on. For adults:
- 30 minutes of moderate-intensity exercise a day on most days of the week.
- To help manage body weight: 60 minutes of moderate-to vigorous-intensity exercise on most days of the week.
- To sustain weight loss: at least 60 to 90 minutes of daily moderate intensity exercise.

If you're on a tight schedule, you can break the exercise sessions up. It doesn't have to be a continuous 60 or 90 minutes. Aerobic exercise of less than 20 minutes, however, doesn't give you the full aerobic benefits. But even 15 minutes can be helpful if you're really overweight to get started without getting breathless. It takes much more energy to walk or do most things that get you moving if you're overweight. A 300-pound person is moving twice the weight of a 150-pound person.

I fall in the last category and on alternate days exercise 60 minute or 90 minute. Just about all the exercises I'll mention in the next section burn about 500 calories an hour, if done at moderate to high-intensity. Research data has shown that while health benefits begin at as little as 700 calories a week of exercise, the full benefits come at about 2,000 calories a week. It's unknown when gains level off.

At my level of exercise, I burn about 3,100-3,500 calories a week. This helped me to sustain an average pound a week weight loss for over two years.[7] Now that I'm at my targeted weight, I've kept my exercise regimen the same, which I greatly enjoy, and allow myself to eat more calories to maintain a stable weight of about 168 pounds—down from 270.

Energy Pathways (About.com Sports Medicine)

Remember adenosine triphosphate (ATP), the molecule that cells use for energy (Chapter 14)? Because the body doesn't easily store ATP (and what is stored gets used up in seconds), it has to continuously create ATP during exercise. The two major ways the body converts nutrients into energy are:

+ Aerobic metabolism (with oxygen)
+ Anaerobic metabolism (without oxygen)

Although these systems can be further divided, most often it's a combination of energy systems that supplies the fuel needed for exercise, with the intensity and duration of the exercise determining which method gets used when.

ATP-CP Anaerobic Energy Pathway

The ATP-CP energy pathway (sometimes called the phosphate system) supplies about 10 seconds worth of energy and is used for short bursts of exercise, such as a 100-meter sprint. This pathway doesn't require any oxygen to create ATP. It first uses up any ATP stored in the muscles (about 2-3 seconds worth) and then it uses creatine phosphate (CP) to resynthesize ATP until the CP runs out (another 6-8 seconds). After the ATP and CP are used the body will move on to either aerobic or anaerobic metabolism (glycolysis) to continue to create ATP to fuel exercise.

Anaerobic Metabolism – Glycolysis

The anaerobic energy pathway, or glycolysis, creates ATP exclusively from carbohydrates, with lactic acid being a by-product. Anaerobic glycolysis provides energy by the (partial) breakdown of glucose without the need for oxygen. Anaerobic metabolism produces energy for short, high-intensity bursts of activity lasting no more than several minutes before the lactic acid build-up reaches a threshold known as the lactate threshold and muscle pain, burning and fatigue make it difficult to maintain such intensity.

Aerobic Metabolism

Aerobic metabolism fuels most of the energy needed for long duration activities. It uses oxygen to convert nutrients (carbohydrates, fats, and protein) to ATP. This system is a bit slower than the anaerobic systems because it relies on the circulatory system to transport oxygen to the working muscles before it creates ATP. Aerobic metabolism is used primarily during endurance exercise, which is generally less intense and can continue for long periods of time.

During exercise an athlete will move through these metabolic pathways. As exercise begins, ATP is produced via anaerobic metabolism. With an increase in breathing and heart rate, there is more oxygen available and aerobic metabolism begins and continues until the lactate threshold is reached. [This is the point where you get a stitch in your side.] If this is surpassed, the body cannot deliver oxygen quickly enough to generate ATP and anaerobic metabolism kicks in again. Since this system is short-lived and lactic acid levels rise, the intensity cannot be sustained and the athlete will need to decrease intensity to remove lactic acid build-up.

Stored carbohydrate (glycogen) can fuel about 2 hours of moderate to high-level exercise. After that, glycogen depletion (stored carbohydrates are used up) and if that fuel isn't replaced athletes may hit the wall or "bonk." Marathon runners may experience the "wall," and for that reason will drink a sugary sports drink. Few of us exercise long enough to worry about it.

Aerobic Exercises

Aerobic exercise, sometimes called cardiovascular or endurance exercise, is any physical activity that uses the large muscles in rhythmic, continuous motions. The purpose of these exercises is to get your heart, lungs, blood vessels, and muscles working more efficiently.

Aerobic exercise should be the centerpiece of your exercise regimen; it is of mine. Many of the health benefits of exercise are attributed to cardiovascular activity. These exercises include walking at brisk rate, jogging, riding a bike, using a professional rowing machine (or boat), doing calisthenics, skipping rope, or even joining an aerobics class at the health club. There are plenty of other options as well.

When I was flying, I did lots of different exercises on layovers. I jogged, walked, and used the exercise rooms that many hotels have. There's also plenty of stuff you can do right in your room with no equipment at all. In the 1960s, there was a very popular program published by the Royal Canadian Air Force that utilized stretching, calisthenics, running in place, and resistance exercises using your body weight, such as, sit-ups and push-ups. I used the program for quite a while. One way or the other, if you have the will, you'll find a way.

Here are the two aerobic routines I do now. Although, as recommended, I only do heavy resistance training or weight training every other day (your body needs a day of rest between weight training workouts), I do aerobic exercise every day.

On the days I do weight training, I do a 30-minute program on a treadmill to warm up and get the blood flowing. I have a True 500 S.O.F.T. System treadmill that allows you to regulate the pace from that of a slow walk, to the speed of an Olympic sprint, and allows you to regulate incline. I start out level, at a pace of 3.2 miles per hour—about that of a brisk walk—and increase the incline, in timed intervals, to 6 degrees—about that of a fairly steep hill. I then take it back down to level, and in timed intervals, increase the pace to 3.8 miles per hour and jog for several minutes before slowing the pace down to cool off. It's enough to work up a sweat and get my pulse rate up to about 110 beats per minute.[8] After a short break, I do an hour of weight training that I'll describe shortly.

On alternate days, I do a full hour on a professional rowing machine. I have a Concept 2 on which I can regulate the row resistance by opening or closing the air vent to its wind turbine that creates its resistance. It also has a computer program that measures pace, distance covered, and calories burned. I work at close to the maximum resistance and cover 5 kilometers in the hour, burning 500 calories. It's a great way to exercise. You get both aerobic benefit and resistance benefit for your major muscles with no impact on your knee and hip joints. If you're overweight that's particularly important.

Mind you, I didn't start at an hour of rowing. At first I could barely do 20 minutes at a much lower resistance. It's something you increase as you gain strength and fitness. The same is true with any exercise.

Anaerobic Exercise – Resistance or Strength Programs

These kinds of exercises involve working specific muscle groups by pushing, pulling, or lifting weights. What we'll talk about has little to do with men and women who work at building sculpted bodies, or competitive weight lifters who lift and push up hundreds of pounds. Although the basics still apply, they're in a world apart. Our interest in resistance training is to maintain and build muscles and bone for good health. This is particularly important as we grow older and our muscles begin to shrink as our hormone levels, particularly testosterone and estrogen, begin to decline. Several years back I was tested and found to have an extremely low level of testosterone. A daily supplement to bring my testosterone up into a normal range has made a world of difference in my overall health, and has helped me maintain and increase my percentage of lean body mass (muscle). You may want to have yours checked.

Here again, if you've never had any professional physical training, I recommend that you join a health club, and hire a personal trainer for at least a few sessions to get you started. Years ago I did. I joined the local Nautilus club that used a variety of equipment to exercise all the muscle groups, and had a free weight section. The club also had a good pro to start us out and answer questions. If you're going to work hard, you need to know how to work smart to get the best results.

I would particularly caution against using a bench and heavy barbells at home. Hand held dumbbells and ankle weights are fine. But pushing up, or bench-pressing barbells, without a "spotter" (someone standing over you to help if you need it) is dangerous. You could blow a muscle or tear a rotor cuff and have the bar come down on your neck and kill you. I tore a rotor cuff once when bench-pressing more than I should have at the club, and needed the help of my spotter to lift the weight off my chest.

Most people don't realize that putting stress on your bones encourages higher bone density that makes our bones stronger. As we grow, older muscle strength also gives us better stability, making us less likely to fall and hurt ourselves.

No matter which resistance you chose, be it your own body weight (calisthenics, push-up, sit-ups, pull-ups, etc.) as I described earlier, free weights, or exercise equipment at a health club or at home, the important thing is to start light, and slowly work your way up. This way you'll see improvement surprisingly quickly without getting discouraged or hurting yourself.

Resistance training is best done in 2-3 sets of 6-8 repetitions (reps) for each exercise, resting for a minute between sets.

I use a Schwinn universal gym that I've had for about ten years. It's not made anymore but there are other really good pieces of equipment available. The good ones run about $1,300. Make sure you get one that allows you to change weights easily, and allows you to do the various exercises without doing contortions. Thoroughly try it out at the store before you buy it.

My workouts run about an hour. I exercise all the major muscle groups of my chest, back, abdomen, shoulders, arms, and legs. This requires 11 exercises, with a total of about 30 sets, and 240 repetitions. The weights I use run from 20-100 pounds, depending on the muscles being exercised. As I've lost weight, I've also lost muscle, although substantially increasing my muscle to fat ratio. Consequently, I've had to reduce some of my weights by 20 pounds.

Isometric Exercise

An isometric contraction happens when there is tension on the muscle but no movement is made causing the length of the muscle to remain the same. This is good for people with arthritis or recovering from joint surgery, because they work without moving the joint. Following knee surgery, my physical therapist had me sit in chair with my heel on the floor and press my knee down. Nothing moves but the muscles contract. We can do the same with just about all our muscles, including our abdominal and pelvic muscles.

Flexibility and Relaxation Exercises

Resistance training basically shortens and contracts muscles. You need to stretch them as well. I suggest picking up a book that deals with the various ways to stretch your body's different muscle groups. Doing it routinely will help you warm up to exercise, avoid injury, and to cool down.

Yoga teaches both meditation and body postures, some of which are quite complicated and difficult. Yoga and Tai Chi both use disciplined slow graceful movements that you may wish to explore by joining a class. My wife took some yoga classes years ago, and has shown me some of the easier positions. It's neat.

To sum up:

- Be smart. Check with your doctor before starting a serious exercise regimen, especially if you have heart disease, arthritis, or diabetes.
- Start slow and light and work your way up.
- Listen to your body—if it says too much or to hot, slow down, lighten up, or stop.
- Drink plenty of water to stay hydrated.

Enjoy. I'm done writing for the day. My row machine awaits me.

Chapter 16

Creating Your Own Wellness Program

Taking Ownership

As we've learned throughout this book, lifestyle choices are the major determinants of good health. And, like it or not, as an adult you and you alone are responsible for those choices. When you think about it, that's the way it has to be. The government can't do it for you. We live in a democracy that constitutionally guarantees us the freedom of choice. Sure, the government can, and should be doing a better job of educating us to make sound choices. And, whether our elected officials politically like using it or not, the government has the power and the responsibility to regulate, ban, and/or inform us of harmful ingredients in our food, as it's doing somewhat with trans fats. There's even a glimmer of hope that in 2008 congress may pass a veto proof bill giving the Food and Drug Administration (FDA) its first real power to regulate tobacco products.[9] Although the bill would not ban tobacco products, it could make tobacco safer and less attractive for people to buy.[10] This is needed regulatory progress, but in the end, if you want to kill yourself by smoking or chewing tobacco, drinking heavily, being overweight, eating junk, and leading a sedentary life, no one is going to prevent you from dong so. It's your choice. You can rest assured that the free enterprise system will gladly sell you the stuff to do it.

167

If, on the other hand, you've decided you want to live longer and healthier, hopefully this book, and the books and resources I've cited, will give you some of the tools needed to achieve that goal. An essential part of reaching it is teaming up with your doctor and other health-care providers to create your own personal wellness program. The major part of what is called "preventive medicine" actually has little to do with others; it's how we take care of ourselves. It's creating a life style that includes not smoking, maintaining a healthy weight, and being physically active.[11] Sure health-care professionals can council us, guide us, and even set an example, but they can't force us to do it or do it for us. That said, there are preventive medical protocols that can only be provided by doctors and other health-care professionals, such as regular physical, eye, and dental checkups, vaccinations, and periodic cancer screenings that are extremely important for maintaining good health.

Getting Started

Since skinny people don't read diet books, like as not you're overweight, and probably suffering from one or more chronic diseases, as I was when I started my program. If you're under a doctor's care, start there. The first step is an overall evaluation of your health, which if you're seeing a doctor, has, to some extent, already been done. If you're not under a doctor's care, you need to make an appointment to see a primary care physician for a comprehensive physical. Either way, your relationship with your doctor, henceforth, will be an important part of your life and is going to last for years. You'll find that today's physicians are largely unaccustomed to requests by patients to partner in a long-term health program. Medicine in the United States is a giant business, a business that makes money by treating illness, not preventing it. And, unfortunately, as the statistics tell us, most Americans are not taking responsibility for themselves, depending instead on the doctor treating what ails them and making them better. As a nation, we're only seeing a doctor when we're hurting and sick. Often times that's too late.

To learn more about choosing and communicating with your doctor, I recommend a book written by my close friend Robert A. Peraino, M.D., *The Consumer's Guide to Medical Mistakes; Information You Need*

Before Becoming a Patient. Dr. Peraino wrote the introduction to my book and helped edit it. His message is clear. Just like everything else in a free market, capitalistic society: buyers beware. You need to take ownership of your own health-care decisions—it's your life and body, not the doctor's—so find a doctor you can trust, and are comfortable talking to and who answers your questions. Be aware that because of the escalating cost of health care, doctors are under a lot of pressure to see as many patients in a day as they can. So, when you make your appointment, state your purpose and make sure to ask for enough scheduled time to have an in-depth discussion along with the physical. Usually doctors (of their own time) will schedule no more than fifteen minutes per patient visit.

Depending upon where you live, you may even have trouble finding a primary care doctor who has the time to accept you as a patient. "The pipeline of primary care doctors has been running dry for several years," said Dr. Barbara Starfield, a health policy expert at Johns Hopkins University. Many parts of the country do not meet the generally accepted standard of one primary care doctor for every 1,000 to 2,000 people. Dr. Starfield said.[12] The reason is obvious. Last year only 7 percent of medical school graduates chose family practice, a field with a median income of $150,000, according to the American Academy of Family Physicians. That compares with $406,000 for gastroenterologists and $433,000 for cardiac surgeons, as measured by the Medical Group Management Association.

Primary care doctors actually come in three different flavors, depending upon the track of their additional three to six years of training after medical school. Family doctors, those that Dr. Starfield speaks of, are docs who treat the entire family, including children and senior citizens. They became very popular as the number of specialists grew in the 1980s and early 1990s, serving as experts in preventive medicine, and as gatekeepers for the specialists. A family doctor's in-depth training for major illness is usually more general than and not as extensive as that of an internist (who treats only adults) and a pediatrician (who treats only children). All three specialties now serve as primary care doctors. Family doctors, internists, and pediatricians all earn about the same income, which is considerably less than that of the specialists, and there's a shortage of all three in many parts of the country as medical school graduates seek out the higher paying specialties. There are some signs that this may be changing.

Physicals, Diagnostic Testing, and Preventive Medicine

Since the days of the horse and buggy, whether you see a doctor for a specific problem or for a routine physical, you'll always have certain things checked—a nurse or a nurse practitioner would do much of it before you see the doctor. They'll measure your height, weight, blood pressure and pulse, and take your temperature. They'll also take a detailed medical history of what medical problems and complaints you have, medications that you take, alcohol and tobacco use, allergies, sexual activity, and anything that would put you at risk for a specific illness or injury. They may also ask questions to help pinpoint depression and signs of anxiety, both of which can have a serious effect on the overall state of your health.

The doctor will review that history with you. This is a great time to focus on your wellness program. A simple statement, something like this, could get it started: "Doctor, I really need to change my lifestyle. I smoke, I'm overweight, I don't exercise, and I feel like crap. I'm going to try and change that. Can you help me set up a program with realistic long-term goals?" Make it clear that you're accepting ownership of that program—you're just looking for help and advice. Every doctor I know would be thrilled to death to hear those words; they don't hear them very often.

Being a physician, like being a commercial pilot, is both science and art. Both come into play when the doctor gives you a hands-on physical examination. Just looking at you tells the doctor certain things: are you morbidly overweight, stable on your feet, do you have curvature of the spine, are you coordinated, do you seem to hear and see well, do you seem to be in pain—a trained eye can see quite a lot. The doctor will listen to your heart, lungs, and the major arteries in your neck with a stethoscope. If you're a drinker, the doctor may palpate your abdomen to check for an enlarged liver or other mass. They'll almost always check for enlarged lymph nodes, and swelling of ankles and legs. Your mouth and throat will be checked, as will your eyes and ears for obvious abnormalities. You may be checked for high blood sugar by a simple "dipstick" urinalysis. It's amazing how thorough a fifteen minute physical can be. It's essentially what my FAA flight physicals were, with the addition of an annual cardiogram and increased vision testing.

This basic physical at my doctor's office is billed at $180—slightly less for young adults who don't require as much exam time. Blood work to check cholesterol levels, kidney function, and other blood chemistry runs about another $100. Most health-insurance plans will cover the cost of an annual physical, less the co-pay. In many plans, however, coverage doesn't start until you first pay the annual deductable, which can be as high as $1,000 to $5,000. Medicare, for those over age 65, does not pay for routine or annual exams. Medicare only pays if you have signs or symptoms of illness. Of course if you do, the doctor will bill it appropriately.

Because of the cost going to a doctor, and the cost of health-care insurance, which can cost over $12,000 a year for a family of four, millions of people in America do without both. About 45 million people have no health-care insurance. As a result, the statistical outcome of how healthy we are, ranks us lower than most industrial nations, despite the fact that we pay more of our gross domestic product for health care than any other nation on earth.[13]

As an example of the human cost of being uninsured, yesterday, after suffering a lightning strike that fried two of our computers and did considerable damage to the electrical system in our home, I learned the reason I couldn't reach Glen, my long time electrician. When I tried to call him, his telephone was disconnected. He wired our new home a dozen years ago and I'd gotten to know him over the years. When asked what became of Glen, Fred, the electrician I reached to do the work, said, "Glen was gone." I naively asked where he went; he often talked about moving to Florida. "No," he said, "he had a heart attack three months ago and died." Elaborating, he went on, "he was on a job and the homeowner told him that he looked gray and should see a doctor." Glen had responded that he was "okay." He went home, had a heart attack, and died. Glen was divorced, had recently declared bankruptcy, had little money and no health insurance. The three or four hundred dollars it would have cost to see a doctor was a stretch he figured he couldn't afford. That decision cost him his life. He was also a smoker and overweight.

These are the same health-care choices we're facing as a nation, and the individual choices we all have to make. As a nation, we certainly have to do better; what we're doing now is not sustainable. We pay almost nothing to educate people and prevent chronic disease, and squander hundreds of billons a year treating chronic diseases and on long-term nursing home care.[14] Individuals and families have a choice to make as well. Make the life style changes to avoid medical bills, spend what's necessary on preventive medicine, or, like Glen, suffer the consequences.

For most Americans living in poverty, the options are bleak.[15] With little money, and usually little education, they tend to eat poorly. The poor usually receive health care at hospital emergency rooms, which do not dispense preventive care. ER care is also wildly expensive, forcing the hospitals to shift the cost to those paying for other services. It's crazy. Every American should have access to affordable, comprehensive health care. Is that economically feasible? Of course it is. We're the only wealthy country in the world that doesn't have some form of guaranteed health care. Americans accept as a fact of life the risk of losing their insurance, the risk that they won't be able to afford necessary care, and the chance that they'll be financially ruined by medical costs. These are risks that would be considered unthinkable in any other industrialized nation.

This brings us to what's prudent for an individual to spend on preventative medicine. The horse-and-buggy physical that I described earlier was recommended as an annual physical by the American Medical Association (AMA) from 1947 until a series of reports launched by the U.S. Department of Health and Human Services in 1984 took a different tack. The U.S. Preventive Services Task Force, a 20-member panel of non-federal physicians, published a report in 1989 that focused on 169 measures targeting 60 different illnesses and conditions. It has been called "the bible" of preventive medicine. It basically recommends that each patient should be treated individually, and it found that annual physicals, as such, were of little value. What brought the recommendation about, in my mind, was simple; the increasing cost of diagnostic testing.

By 1984, the potential for advanced diagnostic testing was almost endless, ranging from relatively inexpensive pap smears, PSA tests, and X-rays, to full-body CAT spans costing thousands of dollars. There are even more expensive options today using diagnostic imaging equipment costing millions of dollars. Because the tests were available, patients would want them and doctors would prescribe them. The more sophisticated high-tech tests are the most profitable revenue sources in medicine. Used indiscriminately, they jack up the cost of health care tremendously. They also can encourage follow-up procedures that potentially cause more harm than good. As an example, a high PSA test reading on an asymptomatic eighty-year-old man might encourage radical surgery, when, like as not, he'd die from other causes before prostate cancer would be problematic. (A PSA test is for prostate cancer)[16]

To determine the actual practices of doctors concerning routine annual physicals the American Medical Association conducted a poll of doctors (specializing in internal medicine, family practice, and obstetrics/gynecology) from three geographic areas (Boston, Denver, and San Diego). They published the results in June 2005. Most of the primary care physicians that responded agreed that an annual physical provides time to counsel patients about preventive health services [94 percent], improve patient-physician relationships [94 percent], and is desired by most patients [78 percent]. (Arch Intern Med, 2005;165:1347-1352)

My doctor recommends an annual physical for adults with medical issues, and a physical every two years for those with no issues. Those being treated for chronic disease or illness, of course, are seen as frequently as required. I agree with my doctor and those polled, that regular physicals for adults of all ages are an important part of a wellness program. While the U.S. Preventive Task Force calls for more talk (counseling) and better targeted screening for diagnostic tests; they unrealistically expect doctors to target these preventive care strategies without routinely seeing their patients. How? The task force also recommends screening tests for men and women age 50 and older. What about young adults? Should they not have routine physicals and be screened before age 50? I think they should. Most of the friends I've talked about in this book suffered or died from diseases acquired as middle-aged adults in their 40s; others, like my daughter-in-law, younger than that.

The FAA's Age 60 Rule

From my work as Vice President of the Professional Pilots Federation fighting to overturn Federal Aviation Agency's (FAA) Age 60 Rule, I became quite familiar with the statistical medical advantages of regular flight physicals.[17] Because airline captains are required to take a comprehensive flight physical every six months (first officers annually), while on the job, we suffer far less chronic disease—including heart disease, which the FAA is concerned about because of the potential of sudden death in flight. For years, arguing before the courts and the congress, the FAA tried to lump us in, wrongly, with the data for the general population. The European Union (EU) viewed the data correctly and lifted the retirement age to 65, years before the United States recently did in 2007.

As a positive consequence of frequent physical examinations, health problems are detected earlier, with better outcomes that promote longer life. And, as the pilot unions have discovered after fighting against change of the Age 60 Rule for decades, if you're going to live longer, it's really important to be able to work at your profession and earn a living longer. I'm very proud to have been part of that effort. You can read much more about it in my book; *A Good Stick; An Airline Captain Lives the History of 20th Century Commercial Aviation.*

Executive Physicals

Many corporations provide an annual executive physical for their top executives. The president and vice president of the United States get theirs, compliments of the taxpayers, at the Naval Medical Center in Bethesda, Md. Most other large and not so large medical centers do executive physicals as well. I checked out the Executive Health preventive medicine program at Johns Hopkins in Baltimore. Here's what I found it consists of—talk about comprehensive! (*Johns Hopkins Executive Health*)

Evaluations are coordinated and scheduled in a single day, with a possible second day if additional studies are reqauired.

- ❖ Medical History/Physical Examination
- ❖ Bloodwork & Urinalysis (includes PSA for males)
- ❖ Chest X-ray[1]
- ❖ Pulmonary Function[1]
- ❖ Comprehensive Eye Examination (Wilmer Eye Institute)[2]
- ❖ Hearing Test[1]
- ❖ Nutrition Assessment
- ❖ Exit Conference
- ❖ Continental Breakfast, Catered Lunch, Convenient Parking & Personal Representative

[1]Recommended on initial and if clinically indicated for return visits

[2]Recommended on initial visit and biannually

Executive Health Fee   **$1,800 - $2,000**

Optional (add to above price range)

Exercise Stress Test	$230
Metabolic Stress Test	$400
Ankle Brachial Index	$110
Body Fat Analysis	$25
Abdominal Aortic Analysis	$185
Mammogram	$585 (screening)
	$585 (Diagnostic)
GYN consult	$200
Pap Smear	$120
DEXA Bone Density Scan	$1,175
Colonoscopy	$1,615
Priority Scheduling Fee	$500
Rescheduling Fee	$250

The folks at Johns Hopkins were very cooperative, e-mailing me the above information within an hour of talking to them on the telephone. My wife is from the Baltimore area where Johns Hopkins is a legendary medical resource she's known from childhood. She and her family participated in one of their many medical research studies years ago.

Another legendary medical center located in Rochester, Minnesota, the Mayo Clinic, was one of the first to offer an Executive Health program thirty years ago. Mayo's prices are about the same as Johns Hopkins, perhaps because they offer more auxiliary services, a little more expensive. Both market to affluent individuals who can pay the toll. Corporations provide it as a perk to key executives, and the wealthy come from all over the world to avail themselves of the services.

The big question is whether they're worth it or not? Two studies cited on the Mayo Clinic's website indicate they are: (Mayo Clinic Executive Health Program)

Study Reveals Importance of Mayo Clinic Executive Exam

The Executive Health program offers an efficient, cost-effective way to maximize a leader's health and reduce the chance of long-term leave related to disability, illness or health concerns. Research conducted in September 2005 determined the prevalence of serious disease and conditions in Mayo Clinic Executive Health patients that may otherwise have gone undetected. The results:

- ❖ 4.9% diagnosed with a potential life-threatening disease
- ❖ 34.4% identified as having a previously undiagnosed, severe condition
- ❖ 47.6% identified as having risk factors for a serious condition

Value of the Executive Health Exam Study

A 2002 study confirmed that routine physical examinations for executives may identify health problems sooner and result in less expensive treatment.

	Total medical claims	Short-term disability days
Non-exam participants	$6,426	4.02
Exec exam participates	$5,361	2.78

Although these studies prove that preventive health care is cost efficient, it doesn't particularly prove that an executive health program is the only or best way to achieve that goal. For starters, the ability of paying $10,000 (including travel and hotel) per initial workup is far beyond the reach of most people. It's akin to paying out $20 million to $40 million to the Russian government to hold a seat as a space tourist on a Soyuz space flight—great fun if you can afford it. For most of us, we can achieve the same goals working with our primary health-care physician. True, it won't be as convenient, and require scheduling separate appointments for testing—and there'll be no catered meals. But many of the tests will be covered by insurance and you'll be dealing with a doctor you'll see again and again—not so with any of the major clinics.

The recommended Screening tests by the U.S. Preventive Services Task Force are pretty much the same as that of the major clinics. Here's what they recommend for men at 50+ (U.S. Preventive Task Force):

- **Abdominal Aortic Aneurysm.** If you are between the ages of 65 and 75 and have ever been a smoker, talk with your doctor about being screened.
- **Colorectal Cancer.** Have a test for colorectal cancer. Your doctor can help you decide which test is right for you.
- **Depression.** Your emotional health is as important as your physical health. If you felt "down," sad or hopeless over the last 2 weeks or have felt little interest or pleasure in doing things, you may be depressed. Talk to your doctor about being screened for depression.
- **Diabetes.** Have a blood test for diabetes if you have high blood pressure.

- **High Blood Pressure.** Have your blood pressure checked at lest every 2 years. High blood pressure is 140/90 or higher.
- **High cholesterol.** Have your cholesterol checked regularly.
- **HIV.** Talk with your doctor about HIV screening if any of these apply:
  o You have had sex with men since 1975.
  o You have had unprotected sex with multiple partners.
  o You have used or now use injection drugs.
  o You have past or present partners who are HIV-infected, are bisexual, or use injection drugs.
  o You are being treated for sexually transmitted diseases.
  o You had a blood transfusion between 1978 and 1985
    - **Obesity.** Have your body mass index (BMI) calculated to screen for obesity. (BMI is a measure of body fat based on height and weight.)
    - **Sexually Transmitted Infections.** Talk to your doctor about being tested for sexually transmitted infections.

A Note on Other Conditions Every body is different. Always feel free to ask your doctor about being checked for any condition, not just the above. If you are worried about diseases such as glaucoma, prostate cancer, or skin cancer, for example, ask your doctor. And always tell your doctor about any changes in health, including your vision and hearing.

Differences for Women 50+

- **Breast Cancer Drugs.** If your mother, sister, or daughter has had breast cancer, talk to your doctor about whether you should take medicines to prevent breast cancer.
- **Estrogen Use for Menopause (Hormone Replacement Therapy).** Do not use estrogen for the prevention of cardiovascular disease or other diseases. If you need relief from the symptoms of menopause, talk with your doctor.
- **Breast Cancer.** Have a mammogram every 1 to 2 years.
- **Cervical Cancer.** Have a Pap smear every 1 to 3 years if you have been sexually active. If you are older than 65 and recent

Pap smears before you turned 65 were normal, you do not need a Pap smear.

- **Osteoporosis (Bone Thinning).** Have a bone density test at age 65 to screen for osteoporosis. If you are younger than 65, talk to your doctor about whether you should be tested. You may need to have this test again after 2 or more years.

Quite a mouthful, but you notice the frequency of the statement, "Check with your doctor." It's from the same task force that doesn't see the value in annual physicals. Go figure.

If you want to check on any specific screening recommendation of the U.S. Preventive Services Task Force (USPSTF), they can all be found at their website (www.ahrq.gov/clinic/prevenix.htm). It lists just about every disease and medical condition under the sun.

Children and Young Adults

I think children and young adults probably have the most to gain from a wellness program and preventive medicine. It's the young that have an opportunity to prevent chronic disease. As we get older many times prevention is no longer an option. The best we can do is mitigate the condition and prevent it from getting worse. Children also look to their parents, who have the responsibility of making it happen, and the responsibility of setting an example.

Personally, I think children and young adults, with or without medical issues, should have an annual physical. It's no guarantee, but certain cancers, caught early by screening, can be totally cured.

For Women A yearly breast exam, pelvic exam and Pap smear can pay big dividends in protecting you from cancer and diseases that can cause infertility. We have a friend who recently benefited from such an exam. A very tiny lump was found by a routine breast X-ray. It was cancerous but caught so early that only the lump and a very small surrounding area had to be surgically removed. She'll undergo follow-up radiation therapy, but the prognosis is for 100 percent recovery. Juxtaposed, her husband, who was also a dear friend, died from prostate cancer several years ago at the age of 54. He hadn't seen a doctor since he got out of the service many years before. By the time his cancer was discovered, he was having severe symptoms and the cancer had spread to other organs, resulting in his early death.

For Men A yearly PSA test and testicular exam can save your life. Testicular cancer is the #1 cancer in young men, and it's curable if caught early. (*Web*MD) As this is written in July 2008, Eric Shanteua, age 24, one of Americas swimming champions is competing in the summer Olympics in China after being diagnosed with testicular cancer last June.

Dental Care

Periodic checkups and treatment are extremely important for dental health. I can tell you straight out, living in relatively poor rural northern New Hampshire, many people do without dental care. They simply can't afford it. There are some state-sponsored insurance programs for children, but they're expensive and don't offer much in the way of coverage (about $600 a year). Medicaid will only pay for one lifetime childhood emergency visit to a dentist. That's it. After that, the family has no further benefits; their only option is the hospital emergency room for pain relief.

The result is a lot of toothless people in the North Country, which is terrible for their overall health. Your mouth is the first part of your digestive system. Your teeth enable you to chew your food into a form that facilitates digestion. If you're toothless, or have poor teeth, you can't chew well, and will tend to eat soft foods such as white bread, and avoid crunchy foods such as hard fruits, vegetables, and whole grain breads. This explains why many people with poor teeth are overweight.

And good, healthy looking teeth are cosmetically important. Frequently, the first thing you notice about someone is their smile. In the past, a healthy smile belonged only to the young. By middle age, most people lost their teeth. Now, with good dental care, improved nutrition, and practicing good dental hygiene at home, it's possible to keep our teeth for a lifetime.

The major threats to our teeth are cavities and periodontal disease. Fluoridation of municipal water supplies and fluoride treatments for children has cut down the incidence of cavities, which has been the major cause of tooth loss in adults. Periodontal disease is an infection of the gums and other tissue that support the teeth. Gingivitis is a mild form of periodontal disease that reportedly affects over 80 percent of adults age 45 and older. The incidence of periodontal disease (a more serious form) increases with age. Close to 50 percent of those ages 45 or older are thought to be affected. (Mayo Clinic Family Health Book 1990)

Here again, periodic visits to your dentist can help you keep your mouth problem free. Proper home care, which is your responsibility, is an essential part of the program. It includes brushing, flossing, and using a rubber-tipped instrument to stimulate the blood flow in your gums. Your dental hygienist will show you how. For most people, home-care alone is not enough to prevent the dangerous build up of plaque that will eventually separate the roots of your teeth from their sockets. When that process goes too far, you simply lose the teeth.

My dentist recommends an oral examination and cleaning by a hygienist every six months for an adult and annually for a child; for those with periodontal problems, such as my wife and me, every three months. Once a year, they'll also take X-rays, and for children give a fluoride treatment. Besides examining your teeth and gums, the dentist will also check your mouth and tongue for any sign of cancer. My dentist charges $80 for a cleaning, $41 for an exam, and $60 for routine X-rays. Juxtaposed, dentures, root treatments, caps, bridges, and tooth implants cost thousands of dollars, depending on the amount of work done. Here again, a stitch in time...you know the rest.

Eye Care

Although there are many diseases that can affect the eye, the three that top the list as the major causes of blindness are glaucoma, macular degeneration, and diabetic retinopathy.

Glaucoma is not a single disease, but rather a group of diseases of the eye. However, the group has a single feature in common: progressive damage to the optic nerve due to increased pressure within the eyeball. It's estimated that over 4 million Americans have glaucoma but only half of those know they have it. Of these approximately 120,000 are blind, accounting for 9 to 12 percent of all cases of blindness in the United States.

Macular degeneration is the most frequent cause of legal blindness in the United States.[18] This disorder most often affects the elderly.

The macular, from the Latin meaning spot, is located in the central portion of your retina, and is responsible for your central vision. In early stages of macular degeneration, small deposits form and blood vessels grow in the macular region between the retina and its supportive layer of choroid tissue. If these vessels leak plasma or blood, the retina cells responsible for central vision are damaged. Eventually a scar may develop, producing considerable impairment of central vision. It's estimated that 1.75 million Americans over the age of 40 have age-related macular degeneration, which owing to the aging of the population is expected to increase to almost 3 million by 2020. (Mayo Clinic Family Health Book 1990 and the Glaucoma Research Foundation)

Diabetic retinopathy, the medical term for a deterioration of the blood vessels of the retina, is a leading cause of blindness in the United States, causing 12,000 to 24,000 new cases of blindness each year. (Mayo Clinic Family Health Book 1990 and the Centers for Disease Control)

The hidden danger is that glaucoma, macular degeneration and diabetic retinopathy may not produce any pain or symptoms that can't be ignored. Risk factors for glaucoma and macular degeneration are: age (over 40) and diabetes, with the chance of developing glaucoma significantly higher for African Americans and Hispanics than for other races. Almost all persons with diabetes show signs of retinopathy and retina damage after thirty years of living with the disease.

My ophthalmologist recommends an annual eye exam for senior citizens or those with diabetes, and one every two years for young, healthy individuals.[19] The exams cost $95. The exams include measuring the pressure in your eyeball (a painless air-puff with a tonometer), and an internal visual examination of the dilated eye.

My mother was stricken with sudden macular degeneration due to stress following my father's death. At the time she was living on her own in Brooklyn, far from our home in northern New Hampshire. One day on the telephone she complained about her glasses. She said she wasn't seeing so well—she was a great seamstress and did a lot of sewing for select customers to earn extra money. At my insistence, she did go to her eye doctor, but not until a week later, and it was too late. The damage to the macula of both eyes had progressed beyond laser treatment to stop the bleeding. She was legally blind; unable to see straight ahead, read or sew. A tragedy, dear reader, you want to avoid.

The week during which this chapter was written I had all three exams; physical, dental and eye. Thumbs up on all! The truth is, I feel great. My internist calls me the poster patient in her practice for weight loss. All three docs want copies of *The Two Martini Diet* for their office libraries. You can rest assured they'll be the first to get them. They've been an important part of my success.

Wellness Programs Work

I didn't invent the term of wellness. Health-care professionals everywhere have come to the conclusion that diets alone don't work and are using the more holistic term of wellness to describe overall health regimens. People struggling to lose weight by dieting alone get frustrated, feel deprived, and invariably gain the weight back. For long-term success, people have to change their manner of living; their lifestyle or, better said, develop a wellness program.

In July 2008, CNN did a story on Lincoln Industries, a Nebraska company employing 565 people. Lincoln Industries has three full-time employees devoted to "wellness," and offers on-site massages and pre-shift stretching. Most unusual of all, the company requires all employees to undergo quarterly checkups measuring weight, body fat and flexibility. It also conducts annual blood, vision and hearing tests.

"When you get the encouragement from somebody to help you with nutrition and to help with a more active lifestyle, it makes it easier to be to attain a lifestyle that most people want to attain anyway," says Hank Orme, president of Lincoln Industries.

The program has been in place 16 years.

The company ranks workers on their fitness, from platinum, gold and silver down to "non-medal." To achieve platinum, they must reach fitness goals and be nonsmokers—and the company offers smoking-cessation classes.

For employees, reaching platinum means a three-day, company-paid trip each summer to climb a 14,000-foot peak in Colorado. This year, 103 qualified, the most ever. And 70 made the climb.

For the company, the payoff is significantly lower health-care costs. The company pays less than $4,000 per employee, about half the regional average, and a savings of more than $2 million. That makes the $400,000 Lincoln Industries spends each year on wellness a bargain.

"The return on investment is extraordinary," Orme says. (CNN. com)

Truly, the day this is written, Littleton Regional Hospital (LRH), which sits two miles from our home, conducted its annual FEEL'N TOP NOTCH Outdoor Expo & Wellness Fair – a Family Event. It was held at the Cannon Mountain Ski Resort in Franconia Notch, about fifteen minutes south. It featured lots of activities, including free health screening, fitness demos, herbal therapies, yoga for kids and adults, free massage therapy, and acupuncture. I know the folks at LRH very well. Be assured, *The Two Martini Diet* will be in their library as well.

Good health, drink up, stay well. Enjoy every moment. Life is precious and short.

Afterword

HUNGER AND MALNUTRITION

When I started working on *The Two Martini Diet* I truly never expected to do as much research on the fundamental components of food, its availability, and where it comes from. But I found I needed to do so to understand nutritional issues. Similarly, when one thinks of malnutrition, one thinks of hunger and the lack of food. I've come to realize that obesity is just another deadly form of malnutrition. Many experts in the field of nutrition have come around to the same conclusion. Inversely, to understand obesity you have to understand the other forms of malnutrition as well. The major difference is that, while obesity is largely a matter of poor food choices, hunger and malnutrition for hundreds of millions in the world is not a matter of choice at all. It's a matter of survival.

Whether you live on a $1.25 a day or less, as the World Bank estimates 1.4 billion people in the world do, or live at a poverty level in America, having enough to eat depends on your ability to either grow of buy food.[20] Either way, that takes money. On a large, commercial scale, farming requires a complicated, interrelated, complex of resources, including tillable soil, water, fertilizer, and expensive, heavy, diesel-powered equipment to plant, harvest and transport the food. Both the equipment and the production of fertilizer, which is essential to modern high-yield agriculture, consume an enormous amount of oil and natural

185

gas. Ergo, as the price of oil has doubled in the last few years, its rising cost has contributed to the skyrocketing price of food throughout the world.

This afterward is really meant to be a heads up—an alert that the world is in and facing a deepening food shortage crisis. It is going to be extremely important that in 2009 the new administration in Washington develop farm, and farm-trade policies worthy of the United States. This has not occurred under the leadership of President George Bush (the junior) and the Republican domination of congress. As the world's only remaining superpower, and a wealthy nation that is one of the world's largest food producers, we have that responsibility. The people in the United States need food security, and so does the world. Starving people are fertile ground for terrorist recruitment—what do they have to lose? This can either be a time of great opportunity to change the way the world views us, or a time of great danger, if we allow millions more of the world's poorest to slip further into poverty and hunger. The choice is ours and history will judge us accordingly.

A Planet of Finite Resources

In the 20th Century, we first got to see our planet Earth from space. It is a globe predominately covered with blue water, less land, and a thin skin of atmosphere. And it's beautiful. I had the joy of seeing it from very high altitude in my career as a commercial airline pilot. It is also a finite world of limited natural resources that has ethically challenged the leadership of nations throughout recorded history. The temptation for powerful nations to take what they want from weaker ones has proved to be irresistible. Historically, it has produced industrial domination of weak nations and colonialism. In many places, we're suffering the hangover from those days today.

In short, resource wars and resource exploitation are nothing new. Its involved acquiring land, minerals and precious metals, forest products, furs, and, since the 20th Century, oil. What is new is that from the drop of the first nuclear weapon on Hiroshima, which ended WW II in 1945, resource wars between industrial nations with nuclear weapons have become unthinkable, even to the lunatic fringe. The concept is called "Mutually Assure Destruction." This however does not protect us from the basic war strategy of poverty: terrorism. And are we not witnessing the ramifications of past colonialism, and past and present exploitation in the millions hungry people in regions unable to feed themselves? I think in many instances we are.

Our planet is fragile: All but the brain dead now recognize that global warming is a serious reality. It's being caused by the enormous amount of carbon dioxide being emitted by the burning of fossil fuels, combined with the methane gas being produced by a world population of over 1.3 billion food cattle.[21] Every world leader, and anyone that has traveled extensively, surely must also realize that the lack of reliable sources of clean, fresh water is a growing crisis all over the world, particularly in third-world countries. But perhaps most disturbing is the effect of deforestation, urbanization, draught, and flooding that is causing erosion of the limited amount of high fertility top soil available to the world in which to grow our food. This, unfortunately, does not seem to be well realized at all. And it urgently needs to be before space-ship-earth runs out of rations.

National Geographic published an extensive research piece in the September 2008 issue titled, "Our Good Earth, The future rests on the soil beneath our feet. Can we save it?" by Chares C. Mann, a correspondent for the *Atlantic Monthly* and *Science.* Over a color-coded map of the world indicating highly fertile, highly fertile at risk, and marginal land areas, Mann writes, "Today more than six billion people rely on food grown on just 11 percent of the global land surface. Even less ground—a scant 3 percent of the Earth's surface—offer's inherently fertile soil (dark and medium green areas, below). Soil degradation can transform production zones into wastelands with tragic speed. "The history of every nation," U.S. President Franklin Roosevelt said, "is eventually written in the way in which it cares for its soil."[22]

Later in the article, Mann laid out the increasing dimensions of the problem: "By 2030, 8.3 billion people will walk the Earth, and farmers will have to grow 30 percent more grain."[23] In order to do this the world will have to not only increase the production of the farmlands already under cultivation, but also cultivate new farmland in many parts of the third world that now produce nothing and have to buy and import all the food they consume at prices they cannot afford.

World Hunger Today

No one really knows how many people in the world are malnourished. The statistic most frequently cited is that of the United Nations Food and Agriculture Organization (FAO), which measures 'undernutrition'. The most recent estimate (2006) of the FAO says that 854 million people worldwide are undernourished. This is 12.6 percent of the estimated world population of 6.6 billion. Most of the undernourished—820 million—are in developing, or war-racked countries, such as Somalia and Darfur, many falling beyond the reach of international aid. (World Hunger Facts 2008)

Undernutrition is a relatively new concept, but is increasingly used. It should be taken as basically equivalent to malnutrition.

Malnutrition is a general term that indicates a lack of some or all nutritional elements necessary for human health.

There are two basic types of malnutrition. The first and most important is protein-energy malnutrition—the lack of enough protein (from meat and other sources) and food that provides energy (measured in calories) which all the basic food groups provide. This is the type of malnutrition that is referred to when world hunger is discussed. The second type of malnutrition, also important, is micronutrient (vitamin and mineral) deficiency. This is not the type of malnutrition that is referred to when world hunger is discussed, though it is certainly very important.

[Recently there has been a move to include obesity as a third form of malnutrition. Considering obesity as malnutrition expands the previous usual meaning usual meaning of the term, which referred to poor nutrition due to lack of food inputs.] (Medicine Plus Medical Encyclopedia)

Hunger and Food Insecurity in the U.S. (excerpt FRAC website)24

One of the most disturbing and extraordinary aspects of life in this very wealthy country is the persistence of hunger. The U.S. Department of Agriculture (USDA) reported that in 2006:
- 35.5 million people lived in households considered to be food insecure.

- Of these 35.5 million, 22.9 million are adults (10.4 percent) and 12.6 million are children (17.2 percent of all children).
- The number of people in the worst-off households increased to 11.1 percent from 10.8 percent in 2005. This increase in the number of people in the worst-off category is consistent with other studies and the Census Bureau poverty data, which show worsening conditions for the poorest Americans.
- Black (21 percent) and Hispanic (19.5 percent) households experienced food insecurity at far higher rates than the national average.
- The ten states with the highest food insecurity rates in 2006 were Mississippi, New Mexico, Texas, South Carolina, Oklahoma, Utah, Louisiana, Arkansas, and Arizona.

Hunger in general is defined as the uneasy or painful sensation caused by the want of food. Everybody at times get hungry—that's the natural mechanism of your body telling you it needs food. When we talk about hunger in America, we're referring to the ability of people to obtain sufficient food for their household. People find themselves having to skip meals or cutting back on the quality or quantity of food they buy. It's the reason more poor people than the affluent tend to be obese. They're more likely to buy cheaper, filling, high-calorie foods, rather than more expensive lean meats, fruits, and vegetables.

In third world nations where famine is widespread, hunger manifests itself as severe and very visible clinical malnutrition. We don't see that in the United States, because, as tattered as our social safety net is, it still prevents people from dying on our streets from malnutrition. But just barely. All our social programs combined, including Temporary Aid to Needy Families (TANF), HUD housing assistance, food stamps, and Social Security and disability benefits, they do not even come close to bringing people above the poverty line.[25] And hunger and malnutrition go hand in hand with poverty. Exacerbating the problem is that food stamps are not adjusted for inflation. Consequently, in the past few years the value of those food stamps has dwindled. The working poor are no better off. Low income wages haven't come close to keeping up with inflation.[26]

The inflationary force of the sharp increase of the price of oil in 2008 on the price of food is expected to drive the price of food up even higher through the winter of 2008 – 2009. In the United States food pantries are coming up dry, and services like meals-on-wheels, which depend upon volunteers driving their own cars, are experiencing a double whammy; in rural areas many have been forced to shut down.

In third-world countries the situation is far more dire.

Why the World Can No Longer Afford Food

Deadly food riots started in West Africa in October 2007 and spread like wild fire into Mexico, Haiti, Pakistan, Bangladesh, West Bengal, India, and Egypt, and have persisted during the first half of 2008, over the rocketing cost of essential foods. In the past year and a half the prices of grains and vegetable oils have nearly doubled. Rice jumped by about half.

Yet, according to Joachim von Braun, director-general of the International Food Policy Research Institute (IFPRI), in Washington, despite the widespread demonstrations, the food crisis has been largely ignored until recently by U.S. and European officials—who pay for much of the world's food aid—partly, he says, "Because no one is starving in rich countries." Similarly, von Braun says he has felt "like a Cassandra" in Washington in recent years, as he tried to warn U.S. officials numerous times that a global food crisis was looming. Even now, he says, "the specialists share our sense of urgency, but it hasn't broken out of that circle yet." (Time/CNN)

As this is written in August 2008, the treat of 100 million more people falling into poverty hasn't spurred the world's wealthy nations into meaningful action. The Bush administration wants to increase food assistance to $5 billion over two years and several countries have pledged more aid in response to the crisis, but not nearly enough. Neither major party presidential candidate has even mentioned the issue.

According to the United Nations Food and Agriculture Organization, there are 37 countries in critical need of food assistance. Many need not only food, but also seed and fertilizer to plant this season.

According to the U.N. secretary general, Ban Ki- moon, world food production must rise 50 percent by 2030. This will require investments exceeding $15 billion to $20 billion a year in the farm economies of poor countries, including research into robust, high-yielding crops suited to poor regions like sub-Saharan Africa.[27]

The experts say that the rocketing cost of food in the world is precipitated by four factors:

1. Poor harvests and trade policies. In 2007 and 2008, droughts and flooding have hit key export regions, including the United States and Australia.
   Following 9/11 the world's richest nations saw the link between hunger, alienation and terrorism. They offered a trade deal to eliminate the agricultural subsidies and tariffs that were pushing farmers in developing countries out of the market and further into poverty. They've all reneged, and seven years later the tariffs and subsidies are still there. President Bush now claims they are not the cause of the crisis.[28]

2. Increased price of oil. Agriculture is an extremely energy dependant industry. Consequently the cost of petroleum and the cost of food rise together. In the past year the price of gasoline and diesel at the pump has doubled. The price of a barrel of crude oil is trading at over $122. A year ago it was trading at $80 a barrel, and that was a record high.

3. Diversion of crops for biofuels. The International Monetary Fund estimated that biofuels—mainly American corn ethanol—accounted for almost half the growth in worldwide demand for major food crops last year. About a third of the corn grown in the United States this year will go to ethanol. Yet at a summit meeting in Rome, the Bush administration insisted that ethanol is playing a very small role in rising food prices and resisted calls to limit the drive to convert food into fuel. The United States wasn't alone. Neither major party presidential candidate has called for a change in our corn ethanol subsidy program.

4. Increasing demand, especially in China. The fast growing economies of China and India are enabling

more people to buy pricier food like fruit and meat rather than less expensive staples like rice. Chinese meat consumption has more than doubled since 1980, and milk consumption has tripled. With such growing demand, more grain is diverted to feeding livestock rather than people. Exasperating the problem billions of people in booming China and India have stopped growing their own food—many now have the cash to buy it.

(Time magazine May 19, 2008)

The world food crisis is a reality. It's partly the result of the great polarity of wealth—the gulf between the very rich and those struggling to survive. In the United States, that gulf is greater now than since the days of the robber barons. It's also the gulf between third-world immerging countries and wealthy industrialized nations. The peoples of each may just as well be living on different planets. Consequently, politicians and bureaucrats find it none too difficult to proffer up token aid packages to countries with tin-horn dictators and fascist regimes, knowing full well that what aid manages to actually reach the people starving is merely a Band-Aid. And we stand by, seemingly helpless, as genocide occurs in places such as Rwanda, Somalia, Darfur, and Zimbabwe. Why? I think because these countries have no oil or any other natural resource we want.

Juxtaposed, since 9/11/2001 we've spent what many think will amount to trillions of dollars engaging in two wars—Afghanistan and Iraq—and in an open-ended War on Terrorism, whatever that means. Many, including myself, think the invasion of Iraq had nothing to do with fighting terrorism, that we attacked Iraq because it sits in the middle of one of the largest oil reserves in the world. If their only resource were cucumbers and squash, we wouldn't be there. And, if we're stupid enough to wind up in a war with Iran, which could very easily involve tactical nuclear weapons, it would be for the same reason.

Hopefully a change in leadership in Washington and a President Barack Obama administration will have the intelligence to change this. (Yes, if you haven't figured it out by now, I'm a Democrat.) The only way the world's wealthy nations can combat terrorism is to defeat it at its root by collectively fighting the abject massive poverty from which it breeds. It's not an easy task, nor one that the United States can do alone, but we can and should set the example and provide the leadership. If we stand by and allow hundreds of millions to stave or go hungry, we'll always be viewed as the enemy, and there will never be a large enough arsenal of smart bombs, cruise missiles or other fancy military hardware to totally protect us.

Alternatives for the U.S. Consumer to Food Grown on Massive High-Yield Factory Farms

One alternative is smaller farms—privately owned or cooperatives—that grow food locally. While this could never substitute for the massive amount of food being provided by the U.S. farm industry, or that imported from other counties, it could be an important supplement of quality foods. This is being attempted in many areas of the country with a great deal of success. Here's a brief look at some of the advantages.

Less trucking and shipping. Statistically the average American meal travels 1,500 miles before it gets to the diner's plate. With the price of diesel fuel now at about $5 a gallon, and almost sure to increase, trucking is a tremendous cost factor. Add to that products shipped long distances by air or rail and there's yet another dimension.

Large scale farms are usually monoculture farms that grow only one food crop over and over again in the same fields. Since the crops are not rotated with other crops, or periodically turned into grass to feed livestock, the soils become biologically inactive and physically depleted. It is expensive technology that regards soil as "support" for fertilizers, plants, and irrigation water. Plants biologically weakened by depleted soil require enormous amounts of insecticides that further deprives the soil of important micronutrients. And both the fertilizers and insecticides are polluting ground water and rivers, creating an environmental crisis all on their own.

Smaller local farms depend on organically supplementing the soil with mulch and compost with crops being rotated. Some, in order to be labeled "organically grown," don't use chemical fertilizers or insecticides at all. Others don't go that far, but don't use as much chemicals because the soil is being otherwise kept up.

Others called "grass farmers" regard grass as the keystone species of crop and rotate field use between food crops and grazing grass fields for animals. One of the showcase grass farms is Polyface Farm, owned by the Salatin family in Virginia's Shenandoah Valley. Michael Pollan wrote a great story about his stay at the farm in his book, *The Omnivore's Dilemma, A Natural History of Four Meals*. (I highly recommend the book.) You can read about Polyface online at: http://www.polyfacefarms.com/

Part of the story focuses on the ethical treatment of farm animals for food. If you value all life, as I do, it's a story you need to read. The factory farm concept of growing and slaughtering animals and fowl produces megatons of meat, but not in a way that many of us can be ethically very proud of. They do it differently at Polyface and everyone seems to agree the meat tastes better. So, they say, do the other foods Polyface produce. Mr. Salatin doesn't ship food. He's against the concept and only sells and distributes his products locally. I tell you what, if I was anywhere near the Shenandoah Valley, I'd be one of his customers.

Mr. Saladin's concept is that the micronutrients in fertile, bioactive soils grow food, including grass that not only tastes better but is healthier for both man and beast. The animals that eat the grass provide healthier meat. I find this easy to believe.

If Mr. Saladin has it right, it could well be that people seemingly eating well are unknowingly suffering from micronutrient malnutrition. The food scientists and the medical community, on the other hand, kind of shrug their collective shoulders and say no, "a lettuce is a lettuce," whether it's grown on a factory farm or a farm like Polyface, and both are equally good for you. They hedge their bet a little by recommending that you take a one-a-day multiple vitamin/mineral tablet and wash all vegetables and fruit before eating.

I think that what we don't know can hurt us in regard to our food supply. We need to know more about the impact of the quality of the soils our food is grown in, and the nutrition they in turn provide us. Need we be reminded that most food scientists are employed by the food industry?

I also think that it's desperately important that the governments of the world use their research scientists to discover better crops and better ways of growing those crops in the poorer soils and climates in the world, including Sub-Saharan Africa and other tropical climates that have been problematic crop producers throughout history.

If we have the will, there are many things that can be done to feed the hungry of the world. Who knows? But for the grace of God it could be you and me.

BIBLIOGRAPHY

The Omnivore's Dilemma, by Michael Pollan – Penguin Books

In Defense of Food, by Michael Pollen – The Penguin Press

Review of Physiological Services, Lange Medical Publications, Los altos, CA 1977

Eat, Drink, and Be Healthy, The Harvard Medical School Guide To Healthy \Eating, by Walter C. Willet, M.D., with Patrick J. Skerrett. Co-Developed with the Harvard School of Public Heath – Free Press

South Beach Diet, by Dr. Arthur Agatston – St. Marten's Press

Fit For Life by, Harvey and Marilyn Diamond – Warner Books

The Zone by, Dr. Barry Sears – Regan Books

Super Size Me 2003 documentary film by, Morgan Spurlock

The Consumer's guide to Medical Mistakes by Robert A. Peraino, M.D. – Vantage Press

ENDNOTES

[1] Your weight [pounds] divided by your height [inches] divided again by your height multiplied by 703 = BMI.

[2] McDonald's, Wendy's, Burger King, Dunkin Donuts, and Starbucks have already eliminated some or all of the trans fat from their dishes. Many hotels and upscale restaurants are doing the same.

[3] FAA medical examiners check your sugar level with a simple urine test. If that colors the test strip high, they then do a blood test.

[4] 50 percent of the elderly who fracture a hip die within one year!

[5] The Role of Moderate Ethanol Consumption in Health and Human Nutrition 1994, Dept. of Viticulture and Enology, University of California at Davis

[6] Juxtaposed, in developing countries almost 1 billion people go hungry.

[7] 3,500 calories is equal to a pound of fat.

[8] My treadmill has a heart monitor that can be strapped around the cheat that sends radio signal to continuous readout monitor. Your target

training heart rate is 50 to 85 percent of your maximum heart rate. Your maximum heart is 220 less your age. You have to get your heart rate up into the training zone to get the full benefits of aerobic exercises.

[9] President Bush opposes the bill and has said he'd veto it.

[10] The FDA could reduce levels of nicotine, eliminate other harmful ingredients, and restrict advertising and promotion to the extent permitted by the First Amendment.

[11] There are other things you can do as well, such as driving safely, using the seat belt in your car, wearing helmets for certain sports, and practicing safe sex, to name a few.

[12] Article by Milt Freudenheim in the *New York Times*- July 21, 2008.

[13] In 2005, the United States spent 16 percent of its gross domestic product (GDP) on health care. It is projected that the percentage will reach 20 percent by 2016. (National Coalition on Health Care)

[14] The United States spends about $10 a day per person on preventive care, less than we spend for the required annual inspection for our cars. According to the National Center for Health Statistics, in 2004 there were 1.6 million residents in nursing homes, costing an average of $6,214 per patient, per month at nonprofit and government nursing homes. This does not reflect the cost of medical care at the facility.

[15] The U.S. Census Bureau reported April 24, 2007 that 37 million Americans live below the official poverty line—12.6 percent of the total population.

[16] In August 2008, the U.S. Preventive Services Task Force changed its recommendations for PSA testing for men. They moved from no recommendations to stating that the age of 75, is clearly the point at which PSA screening of men without symptoms is no longer appropriate.

[17] The Age 60 Rule promulgated by the FAA in 1959, forced airline pilots in the United States to retire when they turned 60 years of age. In December 2007, thanks to my efforts, and that of many others who will never see any personal benefit, the retirement age was increased to 65, matching that of the European Union and many other nations.

[18] Legal blindness: The criteria used to determine eligibility for government disability benefits and which do not necessarily indicate a person's ability to function. In the United States, the criteria are: Visual acuity of 20/200 or worse in the better eye with corrective lenses (20/200 means that a person at 20 feet from an eye chart can see what a person with normal vision can see at 200 feet); or visual field restriction to 20 degrees diameter or less (tunnel vision) in the better eye. (MedicineNet.com)

[19] It's estimated that 40% to 50% of all blindness can be avoided or treated, mainly through regular visits to a vision specialist. (Harvard Medical School - HEALTHBEAT, August 21, 2008)

[20] The World Bank reported in August 2008 that in 2005, there were 1.4 billion people living below the poverty line—that is, living on less than $1.25 a day.

[21] The UN's Food and Agriculture Organization reported in 2006 that rearing livestock produced more greenhouse gas emissions than the transportation sector – 18 percent of the world's entire greenhouse gas emissions.

[22] FDR had firsthand experience with soil erosion. During the depression, vast areas of American farmlands vanished from erosion as a result of poor soil management.

[23] These numbers reflected a 2002 report by the Food and Agriculture Organization of the United Nations (FAO).

[24] The Food Research and Action Center (FRAC) is the leading national nonprofit organization working to improve public policies and public-private partnerships to eradicate hunger and malnutrition in the United States.

[25] You can read more about how our welfare system in the United States tends to lock people into poverty rather than help them out it in my recent book, *Facing Fascism,* available at any bookstore or online at www.Sorlucco.com

[26] Census Bureau average household income statistics reflect a rosier picture because the average is boasted by high-income households that are doing disproportionally very well.

[27] *The New York Times* June 9, 2008 Editorial

[28] In the U.S. large commercial grain farmers are paid so much per bushel out front by the government. These subsidies depress the sales price of the grain on the open market and discourage investment in agriculture across the much of the developing world.

Made in the USA
Middletown, DE
04 October 2021